Oz Garcia is the president of Personal Best, a nutritional counselling firm. He lives and works in New York City. *New York* magazine named him best nutritionist in 1997 and *Harper's Bazaar* has listed him as one of the "Top Ten Nutritionists in America." He has helped celebrities such as Winona Ryder, Donna Karen, Robert de Niro and supermodel Veronica Webb to look and feel their best.

THE BALANCE

The Revolutionary
Supermetabolism Plan
for Maximum Health
and Weight Loss

OZ GARCIA
with Sharyn Kolberg

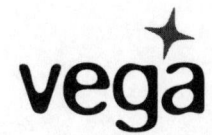

Text © Oz Garcia 1998

All rights reserved. No part of this book may be reproduced,
stored in a retrieval system or transmitted in any form
or by any means, electronic, mechanical, photocopying,
recording or otherwise, without the prior permission
in writing of the copyright owner.

ISBN 1-84333-132-2

A catalogue record for this book is available from the British Library

Published in 2002 by
Vega
64 Brewery Road
London, N7 9NT

A member of the Chrysalis Group plc

Visit our website at www.chrysalisbooks.co.uk

Printed in Great Britain by CPD, Wales

To Clara and Osvaldo Garcia, my mother and father, for the extraordinary and inspiring lives they led and the example they set for me.

CONTENTS

Acknowledgments	ix
Introduction	xi
Foreword	xv

Part I: **OFF KILTER AND OUT OF SYNC**

1: Why Do I Feel So Bad?	3
2: This Test Will Change Your Life	19
3: The Three Metabolic Types and How They Came to Be	31
4: Stressed Out and Out of Balance	43
5: Eating Like Crazy	57
6: Women and Weight: Winning the Losing Battle	73

Part II: **ACHIEVING BALANCE**

7: Introduction to Good Eating	91
8: Down to a Slow Crawl: Revving Up a Slow Burner	113
9: All Revved Up and No Place to Go: Slowing Down a Fast Burner	133
10: The Mixed Burner: Don't Rock the Boat	151
11: How to Live Forever: The New Science of Health	157
12: The Body and Mind in Balance	179

Appendix

A: Glossary of Supplements	187
B: Resource Guide	205
Bibliography	209
Index	213

ACKNOWLEDGMENTS

A book does not happen without the help of many, many people. I would like to acknowledge the following people for all their assistance:

My brother Albert, who has been the silent support and backbone of all our endeavors.

My dear Jan, whose support, understanding, and love allowed me to do this.

Mickey, who got me started so many years ago.

My teacher, Arnold Siegel, for teaching me optimism in the face of great difficulty.

Laura, for all her help and support.

All my clients over the years, from whom I've learned an enormous amount.

My friend, Danny Errico, the best friend a guy could have.

All the people at the Equinox organization, for their enthusiasm and support, especially Livinia and Jody for their constant enthusiasm.

Dr. David Watts, for sharing his expertise on metabolic nutrition.

Eileen Cope, my wonderful agent at Lowenstein Associates, for loving us the minute she saw us.

Judith Regan, for putting her trust in me and this project.

Jonathan Bowden, for his insight and tremendous input into this book. His contribution has been immeasurable.

And special thanks to Sharyn Kolberg, for her ability to translate my thoughts into words, and for her own transformation through this process.

INTRODUCTION

This story begins in 1974. I tell it to you so that you will know how I came to the knowledge I am about to share with you. It also demonstrates how any person can transform his or her life from ill health and craziness to well-being and sanity.

Two years out of university, I was an itinerant photographer working for whichever publication would pay me to take pictures. I ate what I wanted, smoked cigarettes, partied. And I got headaches: searing, debilitating migraine headaches. They had started in my early twenties and went from once a year to once a month, to once a week.

In case you don't know, migraines are more than just headaches. They put you out of commission, sometimes for days. You can't stand light; you can't stand noise. They are often accompanied by severe nausea, and they leave behind a terrible hangover. I knew what migraines did to people even before I started suffering from them. My mother suffered from migraines for twenty years. My earliest recollections are of her staying in darkened rooms with an ice pack on her head. She was also addicted to the only migraine medication available at the time, Cafergot.

So I was frightened when I started getting migraines. I did not want to live my life in darkened rooms. I went to see a highly respected Park Avenue doctor who did a battery of tests; all of them came out negative. "There's nothing wrong with you," he said. The only thing he could recommend was that I take Cafergot for the pain. I couldn't believe it. To me, this was like telling someone whose parents were alcoholics to relax and have a drink. Did he have any other advice for me? The only other thing he could recommend was psychiatric help. Perhaps, he said, the headaches were all in my mind.

I walked out of his office, and the journey through the rest of my life began.

I continued to seek medical advice, but found no one who could help. As so often happens in life, an "accident" set me on the path I was to follow for the next twenty years. The editor of a popular New York magazine asked me to take a photograph of a guru who was giving a lecture on meditation at the East West Center for Holistic Health. I knew nothing about gurus, meditation, or holistic health. I went to the address they gave me, put out my cigarette, and entered to complete my assignment. It was like stepping into another world. There were signs on the doors that might as well have been in another language: Flotation Tank, Acupuncture, Holistic Medicine. As I looked around the center, I felt as though I'd stepped into a Martian landscape. Nothing here was familiar, yet it all dazzled me.

I picked up some brochures and a book they were selling called *The Benefits of Running*. I was not a runner, but the cover showed a handsome fellow running on a beach, and I thought maybe I could aspire to look like that. The next day, I bought a pair of trainers and made my first attempts at running around the reservoir in Central Park. I lasted about ten minutes, but I continued to run every day, and I returned to the East West Center to see what else I could learn. I attended a lecture there on holistic health, specifically about the relationship between food and one's current state of health.

This was a revelation. I cut out my four or five cups a day of coffee. I stopped smoking. I went through terrible withdrawal symptoms and had a migraine that lasted almost a week. The following Saturday, I woke up rested and alert. I was in a great mood. I ran around the reservoir and thought, "At last. I've rejoined the human race."

It soon became clear to me that I had to question everything I ate. I loved fast foods; I loved fried foods. I gave them up. I eliminated all meat and became a vegetarian. I had no more migraines. I became a fanatic. I even lost some of my friends, because all I could talk about was food. But I knew I had saved myself. In 1979, I ran my first marathon in 3:12 and came across the finishing line in the first 25 percent of the runners. I felt I had experienced the ultimate transformation.

At that point, I gave up my successful career as a photographer and went to work at a small holistic health center on the Upper West Side in New York run by Dr. Sidney Saffron. I wanted to learn everything I could about health. Not long afterwards, I opened my consulting practice, where I began to teach people what I had learned about applying the principles of natural living to day-to-day health concerns.

At first, I gave everyone the same advice. I wanted everyone to become a vegetarian like I was. Slowly, I began to realize that not everyone reacted well to such a diet. In fact, I began to have intense cravings for carbohydrates and an almost bottomless appetite. No matter how much I ate, I couldn't fill myself up. I went back to see Dr. Sidney. I told him what was happening, and he said, "You need meat." I fought him on this, but he kept insisting. So gradually I started eating fish and then chicken. And I felt much better.

That was when I began to study the differences among people—why some people could tolerate certain foods and others couldn't. My consulting practice changed. I began to think of my clients in much more personal terms, rather than as prospective parishioners in my own personal cult of nutrition. Despite my good intentions, my fanaticism in one nutritional direction had been leading me off-center and out of balance.

Since then I have listened to my own body and taught others to listen to theirs. I know that people are unique and individual and must find their own way to stay healthy in this hectic world. What I offer to you here is a guidebook: a pathway you can follow that will help you to know yourself and to find the foods, the exercise, and the supplements that will give you balance and keep your life on an even keel.

By following the Balance program, you will naturally have more energy; lose weight; reduce your risk of heart attack, diabetes, and other diseases; feel better emotionally; and extend your life. I changed my perspective and my attitudes about foods, and I changed my life. I run for pleasure. I'm healthy. I get a lot out of life. And I'm happy. The same can happen for you. Try it. Make gradual changes if you need to or jump in with both feet. Just try it. You'll be amazed.

FOREWORD

I met Oz for the first time about five years ago. As I got to know him, I was struck by his intelligence, his broad range of interests and his inexhaustible curiosity. Since that time we have referred many people to each other. As a result I've come to regard him highly both as a health practitioner and as a person. Among the things that I respect most about him is the way he bases his knowledge and approach to alternative medicine on proven scientific data.

Since meeting Oz I have treated many of his clients medically. Many of them have told me how Oz takes the time to educate them and to investigate their complaints. They are thrilled to find someone who listens, who takes their complaints seriously, no matter how "odd" or seemingly trivial. Some of his clients have been treated by mainstream medicine and dismissed with, "There's nothing wrong with you. It's all in your mind," or, even more disturbing, "There's nothing we can do for you."

Oz refuses to accept those dead-end answers, just as he refused to accept traditional medicine's verdict that there was nothing they could do about his own various maladies. He did his own research, using as his greatest resource an unlimited interest in all things to do with human health, and a willingness to listen to and evaluate information from a wide variety of sources. He used what is ultimately his greatest asset: a sharply honed critical intelligence and a deep passion for the analytical process.

In 1997, *New York* magazine named Oz Garcia the best nutritionist in New York. His practice, which was always extremely busy, exploded. The demand for Oz outgrew his available time. Luckily, Oz decided to meet this demand by condensing his 20 years of experience into this informative book.

The Balance is a system of nutrition, clinical biochemistry, physiology, psychology, clinical medicine, fitness, and common sense, written for both the lay person and the healthcare professional.

The Balance is not meant to be a new diet fad. Oz recommends eating based on proven scientific principles and groundbreaking research by standing on the shoulders of nutritional pioneers such as Dr. Roger Williams, who first proved there was such a thing as biochemical individuality, all the way to Dr. Barry Sears, author of *The Zone*.

The Balance takes us further into a system of personal care. Reading it enables you to understand your metabolism and how it affects your health. This book gives you the ability to understand and change eating behavior that simply doesn't work, thus allowing you to control—through food—your moods, your stress level, and your weight. And yes, the right nutrition is the best prevention and protection against many degenerative illnesses. All the patients referred to me by Oz have been successfully educated by him with the principles from *The Balance* for conditions such as high cholesterol, migraine headaches, chronic fatigue, mood swings, obesity, intestinal problems and hormonal imbalances—to name a few.

One "disease" we all suffer from is nutritional schizophrenia. We're bombarded with health and diet information, often contradictory. We end up counting calories, eating meals high in fats and carbohydrates—and then order a diet soda. We're frequently baffled by what we should or should not eat. By applying the principles of *The Balance* and common sense, we can eat healthily without feeling as though we are restricted or on a deprivation diet.

The program outlined in this book is not a diet. It is directed at changing your lifestyle. Oz encourages people to change their lives in order to get the most out of them. He shares with readers what he has discovered on his own nutritional journey, guiding people toward a system of nutritional self-care while empowering them to find their own solutions.

The tools and suggestions in this book are made in that same spirit—not to be blindly adhered to, nor to be taken as the new nutritional Holy Grail. The book is based on the concept of individualism; to take from it what works best for you. You will certainly find, however, that the concepts you do follow will help you maintain a healthier, more energized, better balanced life.

Oz is a healer. I offer my congratulations, *The Balance* is an incredible text that is long overdue.

Lionel Bisson, D.O.
Medical Director
New York Sports and Spine Complex
New York, NY

The author of this book is not a doctor. The advice and suggestions included here are not intended to substitute the advice of a trained health professional. Please consult your physician before following any of the suggestions herein; also consult your physician about any health problems you may be having. If you are taking prescription drugs, do not take any supplements until you have consulted your health professional.

PART I

OFF KILTER
AND OUT OF SYNC

■ ■ ■

1

WHY DO I FEEL SO BAD?

OH, MY ACHING . . . EVERYTHING

"I don't seem to have the energy I used to."
"I feel so run down I can't think straight anymore."
"I diet and I diet, and I don't lose weight."
"I feel older than my years."
"I don't know what's wrong with me, but I just don't feel right."

Most of the people I see in my practice every day don't know what's wrong with them. They can't point to specific illnesses, but they do know they generally feel "bad." They think they should be on a health and fitness regimen, but they haven't a clue as to what to do or where to start. Why do so many people feel that way when health is one of the most talked-about subjects in the news today?

At no time in history has the general public been so blanketed with information about nutrition, health, and fitness. Television networks that used to cover an occasional health-related story now have science and health correspondents with regular daily spots. There are well over two dozen fitness- and health-oriented magazines, and virtually every general interest magazine, whether marketed to men or to women, includes at least one how-to article on nutrition, weight loss, or fitness in every issue. In this atmosphere, we are bombarded daily by new information, misinformation, and study results that contradict what we've been told the week before, not to mention the latest diet fads and nutritional gurus all claiming to have access to the Ultimate Nutritional Truth.

And that search for the Ultimate Nutritional Truth is big, big business. The figures have been quoted so often they've become a cliché: more than 30 billion dollars spent annually on diet and weight loss programs, with a failure rate of anywhere from 90 to 98 percent. In other words, Americans spend a minimum of 28.5 billion dollars a year on programs that don't work for them!

Why do we do it? Of course, we all want to look good. We want to be model-thin and muscularly athletic. But that's not the whole answer. The truth is, we don't feel well. Our cravings are out of control, and our ability to manage them is severely impaired. Our waistlines are growing, our endurance is diminished, our strength is sapped, and our exhaustion level is frighteningly high.

Add to that our twenty-first century lifestyles. We work long hours under stressful conditions. Although some of us exercise regularly, many more of us do not. We have less and less time to shop, prepare, and cook for our families and ourselves. When we do shop, we are dazed and confused by the plethora of foods available, especially by those that are marketed as "healthy" choices by being labeled low fat, natural, and organic.

■ ● ■

Most people who come to see me in my nutritional consulting practice say that their first concern is losing weight. But when we talk further, the list of complaints gets longer and longer. Fatigue and lack of energy are high on the list. Then comes unexplained mood swings, low-level depression, despair, headaches, premenstrual syndrome (PMS), feelings of being run-down, diminished interest in sex, and general malaise. One client reported the feeling of "dragging your ass around all the time."

What my clients, and millions of others, are really dragging around is an overall sense that there is something wrong here and that there must be a way to fix it. All the information available is not helping us. All the diet books, diet plans, and diet clubs are not helping us. We are tired of dragging around soft bellies and loose muscles. We desperately want to regain our sense of passion, of roughness, that "ready for anything" feeling of being on top of our game. We want to live a healthy life in which energy is bountiful, bodies are toned and strong, mental alertness is the norm, and a sense of power and zest are present at all times. What we're looking for, even though we may not realize it, is The Balance.

BALANCED WHAT?

Did you ever wonder why some people seem to do well on a traditional high-carbohydrate, low-fat diet, while others seem to crash and burn on the same fare? Or why some people thrive on a high-protein menu, while others feel heavy and constipated eating the same way? While some people seem to be able to drink two pints of milk a day throughout their adulthood, why do others get bloated and tired after even a small amount of dairy products?

The answers to these questions can be found in the concept of metabolic individuality. Metabolism, simply defined, is the sum total of all the biochemical processes that take place in the body. Our bodies are constantly doing two things: building up and breaking down. These two processes go on simultaneously. For example, food is broken down into compounds, some of which, like glucose, are used to create energy at the cellular level; some of which are used to build and repair muscle tissue; and some of which are transported through the blood to enrich and build tissue. This building-up process is called *anabolism*. At the same time other compounds, like glycogen and fatty acids, are being released from the cells and broken down to be used for energy. This breaking-down process is called *catabolism*. Catabolism (breaking down) + anabolism (building up) = metabolism. When this process is running smoothly, cleanly, and at peak efficiency, we achieve what I call The Balance.

Every individual's metabolism does not function at the same rate. Some people burn fuel at a fast rate. I refer to these people as *fast burners*. Other people, whom I call *slow burners*, have a slower rate of metabolism. *Mixed burners* are those who, under most circumstances, burn fuel at a fairly even keel. The next chapter contains a test (it's simple; you don't even have to study for it) that just may change your life. This test will enable you to find out what kind of metabolism you have. The rest of the book will teach you how to use that information to develop an individualized food, supplement, and exercise program—one tailored just for you.

Not all of the information and diet programs out there are bad for you. Some of them are quite good. However, they are

The Balance

ultimately disappointing because they do not take into account one critical fact. It is a simple idea, but its importance cannot be overstated: We are all unique. Without taking into consideration your individual uniqueness, there is no way to prescribe a food program that will work optimally with your particular body.

Most diet plans are like ready-made suits. If you walk into a department store and you happen to be a perfect size 42 regular, for example, you're in luck. A suit right off the rack will fit pretty well. But most people take that suit off the rack and find that to make it fit—to make it wearable and comfortable and highly functional—it needs alteration.

When you choose a diet program "off the rack," you'll find it just as hard to fit. However, by following the program of metabolic individualism outlined in this book, you'll find out what kinds of foods you do well with and what kinds to avoid. You'll discover what proportions of protein, carbohydrate, and fat work best for you and how to use that information to create meals that nourish and energize you rather than leaving you foggy and fatigued. You'll learn how to time and space your meals and snacks to capitalize on your natural metabolic rhythm and how to make that rhythm work for you rather than against you.

You will, perhaps for the first time, look not just at the fuel you're putting in your body, but at the *match* between that fuel and the particular body that belongs to you. Rocket fuel is great, but not in a Mercedes. This book will show you how to fine-tune the engine that is your body to maximize its ability to produce energy, burn fuel, and lose unwanted fat.

You'll also learn what supplements to take—vitamins, minerals, and herbs—to support and strengthen your food program. There are some supplements that are useful in slowing down a metabolism that is burning fuel at too great a speed, and others that help a slow burner pick up some speed; some that help you deal with specific medical problems, and others that help you maintain general health and even extend your life span.

The third important element you'll learn about is exercise. Just as in diets, fads in exercising come and go faster than you can say "buns of steel." One minute everyone in the gym is straining on the stair climbers, the following week they're sweating in the step class, and a few days later there's a two-hour wait for synthetic rock climbing. The truth is, everybody should exercise. There can be no significant, lasting weight loss or overall good health without it. Metabolic individualism will tell you what kind of exercising is likely to be best for your body. Not everybody responds well to aerobics. Weight training is good for some types, but not for others. Concentrating on the wrong type of exercise can create an invisible obstacle to optimum well-being.

This program of metabolic balancing has already helped thousands regain their health and vitality and maintain their optimum weight without starvation, deprivation, or the torment of constant dieting. By learning to recognize and identify your individual metabolic type, you'll learn to use your own natural resources to turn your body into a lean, vital, fat-burning machine functioning at peak efficiency all the time. *This* is the state I call The Balance.

THE REWARDS OF THE BALANCE

The Balance is designed to help people who, like 99 percent of the clients I see, have problems related to food. Food is no longer seen as a fuel source for survival, but as a frustrating daily battle that seems impossible to win. Having read many of the diet books around, some clients tell me, "I have a pretty good idea of what I'm *not* supposed to eat. But I don't know what I *am* supposed to eat."

After having been fed so many diet myths for so many years, it's no wonder we're all confused. We've been taught that we have to spend less time eating and more time counting calories and fat grams, measuring our food, putting it on scales, weighing it out in little cups. We have learned to regard food as the enemy. We eat too much or too little. We're good when we eat according to some punishing, restrictive plan someone else has devised for us, bad when we cheat or deviate from the diet the slightest bit. All of this has failed to produce the thinner, healthier people it was supposed to produce. Instead, it has produced millions who have an unnatural relationship with food.

When you are eating the proper foods for your metabolic type, you don't have to count calories or weigh out tiny portions of "forbidden" foods. Your appetite will balance itself. You won't be hungry all the time, and you won't have to eat large portions of nothing but lettuce in order to feel full. You'll be able to identify and avoid foods that make you hungry, foods that make you lethargic, foods that make you gain weight, and foods that artificially inflate your appetite. You can lose weight and keep it off without the trauma of dieting.

This is not a program that demands extremes. Many of the clients that I see in New York City are overworked single people who hardly ever eat at home yet are able to adapt their eating habits easily to the Balance program. Those who do have time to prepare meals at home find it even easier. My goal is to help my clients have fun with food. Human beings get joy out of eating; it's one of our greatest pleasures. We should never lose sight of that.

The Balance advocates moderation over inflexibility. It is important to understand that we don't expect perfection. This program is not designed to put deprivation up on a pedestal. When you're eating in a way that is metabolically correct, there is room for occasional indulgence—what I like to call "recreational eating." If you go to a restaurant where the foods are not exactly right for your metabolic type, enjoy the meal anyway and get back on track the next day. It is not "cheating"; it is living.

We make food choices every day. Your choices should coincide with your goals for the day. For instance, I know I have to achieve certain things during my work week. I know I want to sustain my energy and my clarity of mind. Therefore, during that time, I try to stay as close as possible within the guidelines for food, exercise, and supplementation for my metabolic type. On the weekends, or on special occasions, I am a little more lenient, but I always return to The Balance with the next meal.

It's an unnecessary restriction to go through life believing you'll never be able to eat a particular food again. That's not the kind of baggage you want to carry. You don't want or need to put yourself through the pain and strain of believing you're going to be "bad" today, "bad" tomorrow, and "bad" the next day because you're starting your diet on Monday (or someday). Foods that are eternally off limits often trigger major binges; therefore, nothing is off limits as long as you return to the specific plan that is right for you.

Once you begin to follow the plan according to your metabolic type, you will be able to make informed choices. If you begin your days now with a muffin, a tall glass of orange juice, and a cup or two of coffee, you start your day out of kilter and out of balance. But if you have the proper breakfast for your type, you can start your workday clear-headed and energized. When you start to follow the program, you'll be able to make the connection between how you're eating and your performance for that day. When you're in the groove, your daily performance becomes more important to you than what you are about to eat.

Susan, a client who came to me in great frustration, provides a perfect example of the typical diet mentality. A twenty-nine-year-old movie executive who had spent most of her life struggling with a weight problem, she sought my help because she was gaining weight even on a low-calorie, virtually no-fat diet. She was exhausted, unhappy, and predictably very hungry. To add to her woes, she had developed severe menstrual irregularities that she feared would impair her ability to become pregnant. Like so many of the women that I have counseled, Susan was literally starving herself. Though she was malnourished, she continued to gain weight. Her problem? Her diet was all wrong for her particular metabolic type, and no matter how much food she passed up, she would never get her weight under control unless she started eating the right foods for her metabolic type. Susan, like so many millions of dieters, had it all backward:

In dieting, it's not what you don't eat, but what you do eat that counts, and what you need to eat is food that suits your metabolic type.

I designed a completely different type of eating plan for Susan, higher in fat and calories, and lower in the kinds of so-called diet foods on which she had been subsisting. Although she was eating more than she had in years, after six months of The Balance, she had reached her desired weight, her menstrual cycle was restored, and she looked and felt terrific.

■ ● ■

Frank, a successful New York restaurant owner, also had problems with food. Two years ago, Frank was nearly two stone overweight and had dangerously high cholesterol levels. He also suffered from classic "midline obesity": He had a big stomach, a symptom of heart disease to come. Through the years, Frank had gone from fad diet to fad diet, losing weight only to gain it back. Frank had tried the Atkins diets, both the new and old Beverly Hills diets, the cabbage diet, the Five Day Miracle Diet, and the Protein Power Diet, but nothing worked.

Frank's problem was that he had a remarkably sluggish metabolism. It made it impossible for him to burn fat properly no matter what he ate. That's why he was constantly hungry and had frequent food cravings. If Frank was to get his weight and cholesterol level under control, he would have to speed up his metabolism. My prescription: a diet fine-tuned to liven up Frank's metabolic activity, metabolism-enhancing supplements (all are available over the counter, but knowing which ones to take and how to take them is critical), and low-intensity aerobic exercise (the kind that slowly but steadily burns fat). Today, for the first time in decades, Frank is healthy, trim, and fit.

Maintaining a stable weight is just one of the benefits of The Balance. My clients consistently find that this program has produced other positive changes in their lives, including the following:

- Enhanced energy and endurance
- Improved concentration and mental function
- Better ability to cope with stress
- Stronger immune system
- Improved digestion
- Reduced premature aging
- An end to mood swings
- An end to PMS and menstrual cramps
- Reduced risk of developing heart disease or cancer

WHY THE BALANCE WORKS

What makes the Balance program so successful? It is based on the concept that we are each unique, and that no single diet or supplement regimen is suitable for all of us.

For example, some of us may thrive on a high-protein diet supplemented with large doses of vitamin C and B complex, while others find that the same diet makes them grow fat and feel anxious. The difference is in the metabolism. After food is digested, it must be metabolized, or broken down into a form that can be used by the cells of the body for energy. We need energy to fuel virtually every body function, from breathing to thinking, to the very beating of our hearts. Our particular metabolic "styles" are determined by two primary factors: heredity and environment (which are discussed in depth in chapter 3, "The Three Metabolic Types and How They Came to Be").

Metabolism is, in a sense, programmed into us through our genes. If everyone's genes functioned perfectly, and in exactly the same way, we'd all be laboratory-perfect specimens of *Homo sapiens*. But each of us is born with a unique set of genes, some of which function perfectly and others that may be slightly deviant, or "off kilter." When the functioning (or malfunctioning) of these off-kilter genes is combined with the variations in nutrition we present to our bodies, problems are created.

It is this interplay between individual hereditary factors and the nutritional environment we provide to our bodies that produces our "biochemical individuality," a term that was first used by Dr. Roger J. Williams in the late 1970s. Dr. Williams's thesis was that "every individual organism that has a distinctive genetic background has distinctive nutritional needs which must be met for optimal well-being." [*Biochemical Individuality*, p. 167.] It was his belief that supplying the body with the proper nutrients could combat almost any deficiency in the metabolic process that is attributable to defective or deviant genes.

In other words, by *feeding* our bodies properly, we can help prevent many of the problems from which human beings continue to suffer. Many people are under the false impression that the way to cure these ills, and especially to lose weight, is to eat less food. They think that feeling hungry is a good thing, because it means that they must be burning stored fat. But they are wrong. The body does not differentiate between dieting and starvation. When you are deprived of food, your body goes on the defensive—and slows metabolism down. You're not burning more calories; you're burning calories at a slower rate.

In a 1982 article in *Science* magazine entitled "Do Diets Really Work?" William Bennet and Joel Gurin answer the question this way: "Within a day or two after semistarvation begins, the metabolic machinery shifts to a cautious regimen designed to conserve the calories it already has on board. [The body is] determined to hoard the remaining supply of energy pending nutritional relief. Because of this innate biological response, dieting becomes progressively less effective and, as generations of dieters have observed, a plateau is reached at which further weight loss seems all but impossible."

When that plateau is reached and it gets more and more difficult to lose weight, most people give up and go back to their old eating habits. In fact, yo-yo dieting seems to increase the desire for fatty foods. Studies with rats that have been on enforced diets have shown that, given a choice of carbohydrates, proteins, or fatty foods, rats always choose the fatty foods after dieting.

Add to that the fact that the less you eat, the more efficient your body becomes at storing fat. The body begins to produce large quantities of lipoprotein lipase, or LPL, an enzyme that controls fat storage. So when you go off the diet, you gain back the weight you lost and you continue to gain even more weight. This is what causes yo-yo dieting. This increase in the body's fat storage then limits the effects of glucagon, a hormone whose primary job is to help release stored body fat so that it can be used for energy. You have more fat stored than you did before,

The Balance

and it is much more difficult for the body to release it. It's easy to see why yo-yo dieting has been linked to such major health problems as heart disease, gallbladder disease, and impaired digestion.

Following this program can help repair the effects of yo-yo dieting. It's almost as if you have to give the metabolism a slap across the face and a command to "snap out of it!" to push it out of its inertia. You have to begin to re-regulate these fat-inducing hormones so that they are no longer on the feasting-fasting merry-go-round. The good news is that it is possible to start a program of metabolic rebalancing at any time, whatever your age, weight, or activity level.

FOOD: THE LATEST DESIGNER DRUG

Weight loss, weight gain, fat storage, and fat release are all mitigated and modulated by hormones (chemical substances secreted by various glands in the body) and enzymes (digestive juices that cause the chemical breakdown of food within the body). In the past several decades, scientists have spent huge amounts of time and money discovering and developing drugs to help stimulate, suppress, and regulate hormonal output. They have also studied the effects of prescription and illegal drugs on these systems as a way of explaining just why we take, and often become addicted to, such substances. What scientists are now beginning to discover is that food triggers hormonal output just as certainly as drugs do.

As you continue to read this book, you'll learn how the different types of foods you eat affect your body, your brain, and your metabolism. You'll discover why they make you feel the way you do and often influence your thinking and behavior. Following are some of the food groups we'll look at:

- Carbohydrates
- Proteins
- Fats
- Sugar
- Fiber

RESPECTING YOUR BODY TYPE

One of the things that happens when you begin The Balance is that you improve your relationship with your body. It shifts from one of disregard to one of respect, from disinterest to integrity.

Many of the crutches people use to give themselves energy to cope with their daily lives no longer function as biological imperatives. Liquor, tobacco, coffee, drugs, excessive food consumption, and compulsive behavior cease to be necessities because the biochemical patterns that made them necessary begin to improve.

As your relationship with your body becomes one of respect and integrity, other areas of your life, in which your integrity is "out," begin to surface for your appraisal. When you change your basic biochemical pattern it spills over to every area of your life.

For example, a hard-driving type A personality, who never has time to feel how he is feeling, whose motto is "keep pushing," may reevaluate his commitments after following the Balance program. He may begin to reschedule to allow more time for himself and his family.

A slow burner who has built a shell around herself may begin to crack that shell, and long-buried (and ignored) feelings may come to the surface. Things about which she had no opinion suddenly produce strong responses. This is a vital time when self-expression becomes a priority.

The Balance may change you in unexpected ways. It's amazing what you can accomplish when your energy level is consistently high, when your brain is functioning at peak efficiency. These things can happen when you know what your unique, individual body needs—not just to survive, but to thrive.

WHAT TYPE ARE YOU?

The premise of The Balance is startlingly simple: The reason so many of us are overweight, depressed, fatigued, stressed out, and just plain sick is that we are eating precisely the wrong foods and taking precisely the wrong supplements for our particular metabolic type.

The goal of The Balance is to correct metabolic extremes and bring your body back into balance, where it is meant to be. To achieve balance, the metabolism of a fast burner must be slowed down, and the metabolism of a slow burner must be speeded up. Mixed burners come closest to being in balance, but they, too, are at continual risk of speeding up or slowing down if they fail to eat the correct diet or take the correct supplements.

The first step in reaching The Balance is to identify your metabolic type so that you can follow the appropriate diet to bring you back to balance. Take the test in the next chapter and find out what type you are. As you read the rest of the book, pay special attention to suggestions for your metabolic type. It will change your life.

2

THIS TEST WILL CHANGE YOUR LIFE

TAKING THE TEST

This questionnaire has been developed from my own observations, but it is based on a strong foundation of work on metabolic individuality by such notables in the field as Roger Williams, William Kelley, and David Watts. It has evolved over my eighteen years of nutritional practice as an important indicator of a person's metabolic type.

This is not a difficult test. It contains questions about your eating habits, your lifestyle, and your personality traits. When you're answering these questions, don't be concerned with any prior history in any of these areas. Answer the questions on the basis of your current lifestyle and food preferences.

If you don't normally pay attention to your food preferences, exercise, or sleep patterns, take a few days to review them. Observe yourself. Whenever a new client comes to my office, the first thing I do is ask him or her to keep a food diary for a week or two. You might want to do the same. Don't change anything about the way you eat; just record it. Then you will be able to answer the questions in this test more accurately.

If you're not sure how to answer a particular question, go with your first instinct. You might feel that none of the choices fit you exactly or fit you all the time. That's okay. Choose the answer that best describes you under most circumstances. The test is designed to reflect general tendencies.

It might seem that some questions are repetitious. That's because there are always several ways to interpret a question. If a question is worded differently the second time it is asked, it may give you a better insight into how to answer it. Remember that there is no right or wrong answer. We have asked enough questions here to be able to give you a clear indication of which metabolic type you are.

To take the test, fill in the square that corresponds most closely to your answer. When you are done with the test, add up the number of filled-in squares in each column.

	1	2	3
1. *I tend to get angry:*			
easily	☐		
almost never		☐	
occasionally			☐
2. *I tend to get anxious:*			
easily	☐		
almost never		☐	
occasionally			☐

The Balance

3. My appetite is:
- above normal ☐
- normal ☐
- below normal ☐

4. I find it easy to:
- gain weight ☐
- maintain my weight ☐
- lose weight ☐

5. My ability to concentrate is:
- poor ☐
- normal ☐
- excellent ☐

6. I would be more likely to crave:
- bread, pasta ☐
- biscuits, chocolate bar, pudding ☐
- my cravings vary ☐

7. I tend to:
- be depressed or withdrawn ☐
- have normal ups and downs ☐
- seldom be sad or depressed ☐

8. My hair is usually:
- dry ☐
- normal ☐
- oily ☐

9. My skin is usually:
- dry ☐
- normal ☐
- oily ☐

10. *Eating before bedtime:*
    - makes me feel good ☐
    - doesn't make a difference to how I feel ☐
    - makes me toss and turn all night ☐

11. *A meal consisting of mostly fruit makes me feel:*
    - satisfied ☐
    - pretty satisfied ☐
    - unsatisfied or jittery ☐

12. *A meal that contains meat makes me feel:*
    - satisfied ☐
    - usually better ☐
    - tired and sluggish ☐

13. *During the day I:*
    - sometimes forget to eat meals ☐
    - get hungry often ☐
    - eat three meals a day with nothing in between ☐

14. *I experience swelling:*
    - occasionally ☐
    - almost never ☐
    - frequently ☐

15. *Emotionally, I:*
    - have a hot temper ☐
    - have occasional emotional upsets ☐
    - am usually calm, cool, and collected ☐

The Balance

16. My endurance is:
- poor ☐
- normal ☐
- enhanced ☐

17. I lose energy after eating:
- meats ☐
- fruits or sweets ☐
- I don't lose energy after eating ☐

18. I exercise:
- frequently, and enjoy it ☐
- sometimes, and enjoy it ☐
- seldom, and dislike it ☐

19. I fall asleep:
- easily ☐
- within a half hour ☐
- with difficulty ☐

20. I feel fatigue:
- often ☑
- occasionally ☐
- seldom ☐

21. My feelings of anger:
- develop slowly ☐
- develop occasionally ☐
- develop quickly and frequently ☐

22. If I have to choose an exercise, I prefer:
- an intense aerobic exercise ☐
- weights and machines ☐
- either one ☐

23. At a buffet I would:
    choose a little bit of everything ☐
    choose mostly fruits and desserts ☐
    choose mostly meats and fatty foods ☐

24. I prefer my portion size to be:
    medium ☐
    large ☐
    small ☐

25. For breakfast, I prefer:
    dry cereal, toast, and coffee ☐
    juice, coffee, cooked cereal, and toast ☐
    eggs, meat, toast, and butter ☐

26. I get hungry:
    often, with strong hunger pains ☐
    occasionally ☐
    hardly ever ☐

27. My blood sugar:
    is usually low (hypoglycemia) ☐
    is normal ☐
    is usually high (tendency to diabetes) ☐

28. I choose snacks like fruit, cake, or sweets:
    often ☐
    sometimes ☐
    hardly ever ☐

The Balance

29. *I choose snacks like peanuts, cheese, or crisps:*
    - often ☐
    - sometimes ☐
    - hardly ever ☐

30. *My breakfast is usually:*
    - fairly large ☐
    - average ☐
    - I don't usually have breakfast ☐

31. *I enjoy fatty meats:*
    - often ☐
    - sometimes ☐
    - hardly ever ☐

32. *I enjoy potatoes:*
    - occasionally ☐
    - quite a bit ☐
    - I can take them or leave them ☐

33. *I like raw salad and vegetables:*
    - quite a bit ☐
    - sometimes ☐
    - I can take them or leave them ☐

34. *I feel too warm:*
    - frequently ☐
    - rarely ☐
    - hardly ever ☐

35. *My hands and feet are cold and clammy:*
    - usually ☐
    - occasionally ☐
    - hardly ever ☐

36. I'm awake and alert:
    around noon ☐
    whenever I get up ☐
    bright and early ☐

37. I am impulsive:
    frequently ☐
    rarely ☐
    once in a while ☐

38. I think I am unhealthy:
    frequently ☐
    occasionally ☐
    hardly ever; I frequently
    have a sense of well-being ☐

39. Around evening time, I:
    come alive ☐
    gradually slow down ☐
    go to bed early ☐

40. No matter what I eat:
    my weight stays the same ☐
    I have trouble gaining weight ☐
    I gain weight easily ☐

41. My pulse rate is:
    frequently slow ☐
    normal ☐
    usually fast ☐

42. My reflexes are:
    fast ☐
    normal ☐
    slow ☐

The Balance

43. *When I hear an unexpected noise, I:*
    am easily startled ☐
    am sometimes startled
    but not unusually ☐
    am slow to react ☐

44. *My sex drive is:*
    fairly low ☐
    elevated ☐
    normal ☐

45. *I need extra sleep:*
    frequently ☐
    occasionally ☐
    rarely ☐

46. *I wake up in the middle of the night:*
    frequently ☐
    once in a while ☐
    rarely ☐

47. *My mood:*
    changes rapidly upon occasion ☐
    changes frequently ☐
    stays pretty even ☐

48. *My stamina is:*
    above average ☐
    normal ☐
    low ☐

49. *Whatever I eat turns to fat:*
    frequently ☐
    rarely ☐
    only with excessive eating ☐

50. *I tend to worry:*

seldom		☐	
frequently	☐		
occasionally			☐

Total number of shaded ■s in each column:

            1   2   3

      ___ ___ ___

SCORING THE TEST

Add up the total number of shaded squares in each column. If most of the squares you have filled in are in column 1, you are a fast burner. If most of your filled-in squares are in column 2, you are a slow burner, and if you have the highest number of filled-in squares in column 3, you are a mixed burner. The three metabolic types are discussed in depth in chapters 8, 9, and 10, but short explanations of each are included here:

• *Slow burner:* A slow burner releases energy too slowly to maintain adequate health. This is analogous to a woodstove whose fire is too small to heat the room. In a stove, when combustion is incomplete, there is a buildup of creosote in the stovepipe. This metaphor is appropriate for the slow burner's body. Sodium and potassium act as solvents in the body by holding minerals in solution in the bloodstream. When sodium and potassium levels are low, calcium and magnesium fall out of solution and begin to build up in the tissues, eventually leading to arteriosclerosis and/or arthritic conditions. To improve the health status and energy levels

The Balance

of a slow oxidizer, the metabolic furnace (i.e., oxidation rate) must be increased. The extremely slow oxidizer is continually exhausted because of a diminished ability to use glucose (blood sugar) for energy production at a cellular level.

- *Fast burner:* A fast burner releases energy too quickly. To go back to the woodstove analogy, the fast burner is a stove that is burning too hot, overheating the room (the body) and quickly running out of fuel (glucose). While it feels better to be in fast oxidation because of the high energy released, the expense is to the tissues of the fast burner's body: The mineral reserves are being exhausted.

- *Mixed burner:* The mixed burner has an erratic energy pattern: sometimes too slow, sometimes too fast. This is due to a loss of balance between the thyroid and adrenal glands. It is an interim state, generally moving toward fast or slow oxidation.

Your goal is to become a balanced burner. You can't change your metabolic type; following The Balance will not change you from a slow burner to a fast burner or vice versa. But you can become a balanced burner within your type. By identifying your type and learning to eat properly for your metabolism, you will burn fuel most efficiently for your body. You will encounter the state of "supermetabolism" and maintain constant, appropriate energy levels. You won't experience excessive highs or lows. You'll be able to respond to stress by facing problems head-on, calmly, without expending unnecessary energy. This is the state everyone strives to achieve.

MAKE THE CHANGES THAT WILL CHANGE YOUR LIFE

Now that you have taken the test and know what type you are, you can go ahead and read the next four chapters sequentially. Or you can turn to chapter 8, 9, or 10 (depending on what type you are) and begin your program, and then come back and read chapters 3, 4, 5, and 6. Because this is not a diet plan—this is a way to wellness—it is important that you understand the many effects of metabolic imbalance. Reading the next four chapters will help you to understand how you got the way you are. The chapters will help you to understand how stress affects your eating habits, how your eating habits affect stress, and how eating like crazy makes you (and everybody) crazy. They'll also explain the special biological and societal problems women face in today's world. They will tell you how eating right for your body type will help you deal with the temptations, the problems, and the mixed messages you get every day in modern society.

3

THE THREE METABOLIC TYPES AND HOW THEY CAME TO BE

ONE HUNDRED THOUSAND YEARS OF EATING HABITS

Like everything else in the modern world, the eating habits of humans have evolved over the last hundred thousand years. Unlike most other evolutionary changes in the world, however, our eating habits may not lead to the survival of the fittest. In fact, these habits may be leading to the extinction of the fattest.

Early humans were not fat. Their diet was determined by what they could kill with primitive weapons, or what they could find on the ground or pick from climbable trees. There were no dairy products, yet humans in Paleolithic times showed no signs of osteoporosis. There was no agriculture—hence no wheat or wheat products—yet prehistoric people were comparatively healthy. Their life span may have been shorter than ours, but that was generally because life was much harder. Humans died from exposure to extreme weather, from becoming prey to the very animals they hunted, from succumbing to infectious diseases. They did not die from heart disease, lung cancer, or high blood pressure.

In a 1985 article in the *Wall Street Journal*, Harvard University anthropologist Irven DeVore stated, "We were vaulted into the 20th century with the heart, mind and body of a hunter-gatherer." In fact, there has been little genetic evolution of humans in the last hundred thousand years.

The nutritional needs and habits of early humans, carried in the genes for all these generations, still affect the ways that we eat. According to Professor DeVore, the food available to cave dwellers was low in sodium. Sodium is an essential mineral that helps regulate the distribution of fluids within the body and is involved (along with potassium) in muscle contraction and expansion as well as in nerve stimulation. Because it was not readily available, humans evolved a craving for salt. Because cave dwellers were so physically active, they needed fat (rare in hunted game) and fruit sugars to provide energy. Cravings for these nutrients evolved to provide the impetus for humans to search them out, ensuring survival. These cravings then became embedded in the genes, which is why we continue to crave these nutrients today.

ADAPTING FOR SURVIVAL

Homo sapiens is a highly adaptive animal. As early humans migrated from Africa into areas both north and south, their bodies adapted to life in ecologically diverse climates so that they could survive on the foods that were available. For instance, people who migrated from Eastern Europe (across what is now the Bering Strait) into Alaska evolved the capacity to survive on diets consisting mainly of hunted game and fish. That means that 80 percent or more of Eskimos' calories come from meat and fat. Current wisdom holds that Eskimos should be suffering from clogged arteries and dying of heart attacks at alarming rates. Yet studies have shown that Eskimos have hardly any heart disease and show few signs of elevated triglycerides or cholesterol.

At the other extreme of geography and climate were people who migrated south to the Indian continent. Those people evolved to survive on little, if any, animal protein. Their diet consisted almost entirely of fruits and vegetables. They even evolved an intrinsic factor that allowed them to synthesize vitamin B12 (which we normally get from animal protein and animal products such as milk, cheese, and eggs) in their systems.

What I have described is the evolution of two radically different metabolic types: efficient meat eaters and efficient vegetarians. These are examples of human adaptivity being pushed along by climate, environment, and regionally available food sources. These two peoples have become so strongly adapted that if they move out of their environment and make changes in their diet, their health and well-being are profoundly affected, usually not for the better.

Most people, however, don't fall into one extreme category or another. We tend to fall somewhere in between, with one metabolic type being dominant. We are, in fact, one of the few omnivorous animal species, with an enormous capacity for variety in what we eat.

BE CAREFUL WHAT YOU WISH FOR . . .

Since the time the cave dwellers roamed the earth, human beings have wished for an abundance of food. And since those cave dwelling times, the quest for abundance has both helped and harmed the human species. When the Cro-Magnons learned better and more efficient ways to hunt, about 40,000 B.C., they soon all but eliminated the very animals they depended on for survival, decimating the big game that was their major food source.

Beginning approximately ten to twelve thousand years ago, several factors combined to change the way humans ate. Owing to a rapidly expanding human population, many of the game meats early humans depended on became much more difficult to find, if not altogether extinct. Climatic changes wiped out some of the plant life previously available. Agriculture and the domestication of animals for food became the main sources of the diet of *Homo sapiens*. We did not change our eating habits because our bodies were evolving differently. We changed our eating habits because the foods that were abundant earlier were abundant no more.

These changes in the availability of food sources forced humans to migrate out of Africa. Dr. Peter J. D'Adamo has done extensive research on human ancestry, migration, and the development of blood types. Dr. D'Adamo theorized that in the beginning there was only one blood type; according to him, all Cro-Magnons were blood type O. When migration began toward Asia and the Middle East between 25,000 and 15,000 B.C., the human diet changed radically.

"The cultivation of grains and livestock changed everything," says Dr. D'Adamo in the book *Eat Right for Your Type*. Drastic alterations in Neolithic people's diet and environment "resulted in an entirely new mutation in the digestive tracts and the immune systems . . . that allowed them to better tolerate and absorb cultivated grains and other agricultural products. Type A was born."

When humans migrated into Eastern Europe, blood type B evolved. Type AB blood, the rarest and most recent blood type, came from the intermingling of Caucasians and Mongolians approximately twelve hundred years ago.

Humans adapted to the types of food that were found, or that could be produced, in the regions in which they settled. The quest for an abundance of food continued in all these regions. In modern times, many regions of the world (especially first world countries such as the United States and much of Europe) have produced that abundance, facilitated by the advent of industrial technologies, including the railroad, the automobile, and the eighteen-wheeler, and methods of food preservation such as refrigeration. These inventions and innovations allow industrialized countries to provide nonlocal, nonseasonal foods to human beings at any time of the year. As humans moved forward in time, closer to the twentieth century, the foods we ate no longer had any relationship to the evolutionary requirements of our different metabolic types.

We evolved to want what we need. We need vitamin C, so we crave sweet things. But the food choices we make no longer represent the things in the environment that are necessary for our survival. The craving for vitamin C is no longer connected to the sweet fruit we had to climb a tree to get, but to the gourmet ice cream we get at the supermarket. The salt our bodies need is no longer satisfied by salty game meat, but by processed snacks found in the local shop. Cravings that were originally satisfied by foods that helped us survive are now satisfied by foods that are killing us bite by bite.

Dr. Patrick Quillin, in his book *Health Nutrients*, coined the term "factory specification diet." He used the term to refer to the particular dietary needs of each species. For instance, the factory specification diet for a cow is grass, and for a squirrel, it is nuts. If a cow or a squirrel were fed meat or fish, it could not go on living a healthy life.

Dr. Quillin compared primitive people's diet to modern people's and found us sorely lacking. His findings show that in primitive people, the ratio of polyunsaturated to saturated fat was about 3:1. In modern humans, that ratio is 1:3. Dr. Quillin goes on to say that "there is a 9-fold deterioration in the factory specifications of fat intake alone. These early primitives consumed 16 times more potassium than sodium. We consume 4 times more sodium than potassium. That's a 6,400 percent deterioration in this critical balance of electrolytes. ... These primitives ate 10 times the vitamin C and six times the fiber than the average American consumes."

What we have now are broad mismatches between what is currently available for people to eat and what we need as individual metabolic types.

Take two different scenarios. In the first, we are taking a cross-country journey from New York to California. What we would like to find along the way are restaurants that serve hormone-free poultry or fresh fish, salads with a great variety of raw greens, and vegetables that are grown locally and served freshly cooked. We'd like to be able to find a wide variety of healthy offerings, depending on what part of the country we're in at the moment.

Instead, what we find on our long journey are fast foods, products of a culture that is driven by expedience. The only variety we get is when we have a quick-cooked pizza (with extra cheese and sausage) for lunch and a fat-filled burger (with fries and a chocolate shake) for dinner.

The second scenario is one we find in the large cities and, more and more often, in smaller cities as well. These cities are home to many different types of people who all live in the same geographical area: human beings in all sizes, shapes, races, and colors. All these different types, with various ancestry and medical histories, live together in an artificial construct: the city itself. The ethnic diversity found in such cities demands that a huge variety of foods be available at all times. So we have "unnatural" food sources available in abundance year-round.

For example, in a northern city like New York, tropical fruits are available throughout the year. Biologically, when winter arrives and it's –7 degrees outside, the body should be adapting itself to deal with dramatic drops in temperature by eating foods that tend to produce heat. What happens when we then feed it tropical fruit, a food extremely high in sugar? What is the effect on the body's metabolism? What is the effect on craving? What is the effect on the immune system? Tropical fruits tend to cool bodies down. When we consume oranges, grapefruit, and pineapple (or their juice) in the winter, even though they're good sources of vitamin C they have a depressing effect on the immune system. It's a poor metabolic match, and it counters what evolution has determined to be healthy for us.

In the quest for abundance and variety, modern-day humans have also lessened the medicinal and therapeutic aspects of food. We use preservatives that make our foods last longer but reduce their vitamin content. Instead of eating whole grains, we process grain into white flour and white flour products. We produce a white crystalline chemical known as sugar, then combine it with highly processed white flour so that we can prepare baked goods that appeal to our ever-more demanding palates.

We consume these foods in outrageous amounts. In the UK and USA, around half the total population is overweight, and studies have shown that one in four Americans and around one in five British people are clinically obese. And we are steadily gaining. In the UK, the average woman is 9lb/4kg heavier now than in 1980. This is one of the reasons we have seen a dramatic rise in degenerative illnesses in the Western world: arteriosclerosis, cancer, elevated cholesterol, problems of the lower bowel, and diabetes. The refined foods that we continue to eat in huge portions were not part of the human evolutionary food chain. They have been created for mass appeal and consumption, and are designed in large part for their entertainment value, not their nutrient value.

WHAT DO WE DO NOW?

As you can see, modern humans are a product of the past. If we want to understand our present, we need only look back to our earliest ancestors, who roamed the savannahs and grasslands grazing on fruits, vegetables, legumes, and nuts. They were vegetarians, and their high-carbohydrate diet was broken down by the body fairly rapidly. As a result, these early humans developed a metabolic type that works efficiently on a vegetarian diet.

Our ancestors who lived in cold climates, where fruits and vegetables were scarce, found fatty meats abundant. These carnivorous relatives of ours developed a slower metabolism, because breaking down fat takes longer than breaking down carbohydrates.

Still others of our ancestors lived in more temperate climates, where meat and vegetable foodstuffs were available, and they developed a metabolism that could accommodate their hybrid diet.

Thousands of years have passed, but we still carry the genetic codes of our ancestors. People may be created in a broad range of colors, shapes, and sizes, but we can all fit into one of the three general metabolic types: fast, slow, and mixed. Understanding which type you are is the key to understanding which foods you should eat, what supplements you should take, and what type of exercise plan you should follow to improve your overall health, lose weight, and achieve The Balance.

You took the test in the last chapter, so you have an idea of what metabolic type you are, and now you have a better understanding of how that type came to be. You can use that information to structure an eating and exercise program that's right for your metabolic type. As a consequence, you'll begin to move away from eating habits that have made you feel progressively less energetic and have contributed to inexplicable illnesses, weight gain, and a metabolic imbalance. By following the Balance program and eating the foods most suitable for your type, you can correct that imbalance.

Most diet books and prescriptions, including guidelines put out by the government, contain nutritional recommendations made on the basis of what the authors think is best for most of the people most of the time. But you are not most people. You are an individual, and by paying attention to your own individuality, you can discover a way of eating that may not be right for everyone else but is going to work best for you.

One of the recommendations that is currently being made both in diet books and in the government's current guidelines is that people eat fairly large amounts of carbohydrates. Historically, humans have never had as many carbohydrates in their diet as we do today. The only civilization to come close was that of the early Egyptians. Because of the large number of mummies left behind and the in-depth analysis of mummified remains that has occupied scientists for many years, much is known about this culture. There are also libraries of written history, in the form of papyrus fragments, that the Egyptians left behind, describing their lifestyles in great detail.

Ancient Egypt appears to be the only early culture in which high volumes of carbohydrates were consumed, including wheat flour, which was baked into bread. It is not surprising that there were many similar health problems to those we have today. Scientists have found evidence of obesity, heart disease, and rotting teeth in similar proportions to those found in modern, first world cultures.

When you think of all the carbohydrates you eat every day, do you include breads, grains, and pastas? Do you include cakes and pies? Fruits and vegetables? These are all carbohydrates. Carbohydrates include all starches, grains, grain products, root vegetables, and fruits, as well as their products and derivatives. Sugars are known as simple carbohydrates, which are readily digestible. Starches are complex carbohydrates; they require a longer time for digestion because they must be broken down by enzymes into simple sugars. Complex carbohydrates are made up of chains of simple sugars.

You could be in trouble if you are consuming a large proportion of the wrong kind of carbohydrates in your diet. I discuss the problems associated with eating too many carbohydrates in detail in chapter 5, "Eating Like Crazy."

My point here is that our current eating habits have made certain foods predominant in our diet, foods that not only don't suit our individual metabolic types, but don't suit us well as human beings. The consequence is that the imbalances in our food sources tend to amplify the imbalances of our individual metabolic types. Both slow and fast burners have certain metabolic imbalances built in, and the foods most people eat only make those imbalances worse. Mixed burners, who are generally better balanced, can easily throw themselves off kilter by eating the wrong foods.

HOW THE METABOLIC SYSTEM WORKS

The Balance program is concerned with the efficiency of the energy-producing systems within the body. Energy is produced by the neural (or nerve) and endocrine (or hormonal) systems of the body, specifically the sympathetic and parasympathetic nervous systems, the adrenal and thyroid glands, and the parathyroid glands and pancreas. Whether you are a fast or slow burner depends on which of these systems and hormone producers dominates your metabolism.

Fast burners are dominated by the adrenal system and the thyroid gland. The adrenal system and thyroid gland are, in turn, dominated by the sympathetic nervous system, which is part of the autonomic, or involuntary nervous system. The involuntary nervous system controls basic bodily functions like heart rate, respiration, blood pressure, hormonal balance, and metabolism. The sympathetic nervous system is associated with stimulatory hormones such as adrenaline and cortisol. When the sympathetic nervous system is active, the heart rate is elevated and the body experiences increases in circulation, oxygen supply, metabolism, and energy. The sympathetic nervous system goes into overdrive when a threatening or arousing situation occurs.

Slow burners, on the other hand, are dominated by the parathyroid gland and the pancreas, which are in turn dominated by the parasympathetic nervous system (which is also part of the involuntary nervous system). The parasympathetic nervous system is associated with sedating hormones such as calcitonin. When the parasympathetic system is active, the heart rate slows down, and the body experiences decreases in oxygen supply, metabolism, and energy. The sympathetic and parasympathetic systems work together to keep us on an even keel.

Suppose you are walking down a darkened street one night, and you see a figure approaching. The figure looks slightly menacing, and you know there have recently been robberies in this neighborhood. Your sympathetic nervous system goes into high gear. Adrenaline and cortisol are released to bring you to a heightened state of awareness and alarm. The sympathetic nervous system stimulates the release of sugar to get your blood pressure up. Your nerves are on edge, and you're ready to respond to the fight-or-flight reflex. As the figure comes closer, you realize it is only old Mr. Jones wearing a hooded jacket. But your heart is still beating rapidly and you're breathing hard. Now the parasympathetic nervous system does its job: It kicks in the sedating hormones that will reregulate and calm the system down.

In fast burners, the sympathetic nervous system is always "on." They are often what we call type A personalities: overachievers who tend to be overactive and have a difficult time relaxing. Slow burners are more often type B personalities. They are not as frenetic and are much slower to become anxious, angry, or agitated.

When you find yourself in a stressful situation, your hormones kick in, no matter which metabolic type you are. It's a matter of degree. In the next chapter, I discuss how stress affects each of the metabolic types and how, by using the principles of The Balance, you can overcome its adverse effects on your immune and cardiovascular systems, as well as on your emotional life.

4

STRESSED OUT AND OUT OF BALANCE

STRESS: YOU CAN'T LIVE WITH IT, YOU CAN'T LIVE WITHOUT IT

We've all seen those movies in which a type A personality—the driven, insensitive workaholic company head—works himself into such a state that his heart finally rebels and "attacks" him when he is at the pinnacle of his career. Another corporate executive bites the dust. He couldn't take the stress anymore.

Those movies may be melodramatic, but they are based on a truth of life. Stress kills. It doesn't always come in the form of a heart attack. Stress affects not only our cardiovascular system, but also our immune system, our nervous system, our digestive system, and our overall state of physical and emotional well-being. The effects of stress aren't ephemeral or abstract, or only in our minds. Stress creates tangible biological and neurological changes that drastically upset the body's metabolic balance.

Stress is usually defined as any stimulus that disturbs or interferes with the normal physiological equilibrium of an organism. Stress can occur through fear or pain, but it can also occur when one is overstimulated by "too much of good thing." Stress can cause disease, but it can also be caused *by* disease. It can cause metabolic imbalances, and it can be caused *by* metabolic imbalances.

It's almost impossible to pinpoint exactly what constitutes stress. The old saying "one man's meat is another man's poison" definitely applies here. Stress is different for everyone. Some people (mostly fast burners) thrive on stress. Stress is their prime motivator; they usually juggle several projects at once and function best when the deadline is closest. These people seem to have a heightened capacity to deal with stress. Others (mostly slow burners) prefer to handle life at a slower pace, one thing at a time, with no unnecessary distractions.

THE STAGES OF STRESS

We cannot always avoid the distractions that life presents. However, the better we understand stress and how it affects our bodies, the better we can learn to cope. First, we should note that stress is not necessarily a bad thing. Some types of stress can be motivating and positive; many people learn to use stress to their advantage. People who are constantly in high-stress, high-pressure situations, such as actors, professional athletes, and politicians, know that the adrenaline rush that comes from being in a stressful situation can give them that energy, that feeling of being on the edge and at the top of the game. If you are a person who reacts positively to stress, and your opponent is not, you have an immediate edge.

Human beings are constantly under stress. It is both inescapable and indispensable to life. If there is no stress, there is no life. It's only when the stress becomes distress, when it becomes intense and prolonged, that it can be destructive to the body and can lead to physical deterioration.

In 1956, Dr. Hans Selye wrote *The Stress of Life*, the seminal book on the subject. In it, he described stress as "the nonspecific response of the body to any demand made upon it" and called this response the general adaptation syndrome (GAS). The GAS consists of three stages:

1. The alarm reaction: a "call to arms" of our defensive forces
2. The resistance stage: fighting off the stress
3. The exhaustion stage: succumbing to the stress

In 1990, Dr. David Watts, author of *Trace Elements and Other Essential Nutrients*, added two more stages to the GAS, as follows:

1. The alarm reaction
2. The resistance stage
3. The recovery stage
4. The adaptation stage
5. The exhaustion stage

When you were walking down that dark street, as depicted in the last chapter, and you saw a menacing figure approaching, your alarm reaction went into high gear. The sympathetic, or involuntary, nervous system sent off a signal, notifying the neuroendocrine and immune systems of an assault. This is what brings on the fight-or-flight response.

During this stage, the sympathetic nervous system works overtime, which results in a high metabolic rate. This in turn results in the loss of certain essential minerals, such as calcium and magnesium. The body may also use up its store of certain vitamins, causing deficiencies to develop. The longer the stress remains, the better the chances that nutritional problems and deficiencies will result.

During this alarm reaction, the adrenal system responds by secreting adrenaline and cortisol. Your heart rate goes up. You can feel it pounding in your chest. Your lungs take in more oxygen in order to fuel your muscles should flight be necessary. You move into a state of readiness to deal with attack. Suppose a predator really is coming toward you. You respond by moving rapidly, supported by the excess adrenaline and energy, to get out of harm's way.

As you're running, you go into the resistance stage. You start to think, to be aware of your surroundings. You recognize the source of your alarm. You realize you can't just run in any direction, you need to look for shelter, or help, or a way out of the situation. The body's metabolism is still high, but it is returning to a more normal level. However, if this stage continues for a long period of time, you can get into trouble. The adrenal glands are drawing energy and nutrients from reserves elsewhere in the body.

If you've found shelter or help or a way out, you go into the recovery stage. Most stressful situations end here. The problem is solved, the predator is beaten, and your metabolism returns to normal. But suppose the predator is only temporarily beaten. You know that it will return, but you don't know when. You're always looking over your shoulder, waiting for its return. You then go into the adaptation stage.

This is when differences in personalities come in. Hans Selye identified two types of stress: *distress* (the word comes from the Latin *dis*, which means bad) and *eustress* (from the Greek *eu*, which means good). Whether the stress is positive or negative, the body has the same response. However, in his book *The Stress of Life* Selye wrote, "The fact that eustress causes much less damage than distress graphically demonstrates that it is 'how you take it' that determines, ultimately, whether one can adapt successfully to change."

If you are someone who can "take it" well, you will prepare yourself both physically and mentally for the predator's possible return. You'll be like the third little pig, who wisely built his house of bricks to keep the wolf away. If you don't "take it" well, you will not-so-wisely build your house of straw and spend most of your time worrying about the predator's possible return. You may end up with what Selye described as "diseases of adaptation" like ulcers and heart disease.

If stress becomes extremely intense and continuous, the body will exhaust itself. The reserves the body was calling on in the resistance stage will dry up, and the body will give out owing to an inability to recover or adapt to the stress. You succumb, collapse, and unfortunately are done in by the predator.

These stages of stress are a normal reaction by the body. Usually, we progress relatively rapidly from the alarm stage to the recovery stage. However, we sometimes get stuck in one stage. If that occurs, disease may result. In fact, it has been estimated that up to 80 percent of all illnesses are now caused by stress-related disorders. These diseases range from migraine headaches, high blood pressure, ulcers, arthritis, asthma, and eczema to eating disorders and heart disease. In his book *Trace Elements and Other Essential Nutrients*, Dr. David Watts explains how (among other conditions) arthritis and gastritis may develop if the alarm stage develops and does not proceed to the resistance stage. Extensive destruction can occur throughout the body, and degenerative diseases, even cancer, can develop in the resistance stage. According to Watts, "[then] the recovery stage is hopefully reached and is the last stage of the stress reaction. However, if a severe nutritional imbalance occurs, then a person may not recover, but instead may go into an exhaustion stage."

If this happens, it becomes imperative to get the body back into metabolic balance. There are warning signs that stress is building up to the danger point. Some of them include:

- Frequent or constant irritability
- Inability to concentrate
- Feelings of weakness or dizziness
- Chronic fatigue
- Insomnia
- Grinding of the teeth
- Free-floating anxiety
- Chronic digestive problems
- PMS
- Lower back or neck pain
- A change in eating habits—eating either too much or too little
- Increased use of stimulants such as caffeine, tobacco, drugs, or alcohol
- Frequent accidents

STRESS IN THE MODERN WORLD

The stress response, like our cravings for sweets and salt, was developed as part of our evolutionary survival skills. If we did not get that surge of adrenaline and buildup of energy in the alarm stage, we might not be able to escape danger. These responses came about so that we could survive in a hostile environment. One hundred thousand years later, we still have the physiological and neurological responses of a hunter-gatherer. The same adrenaline and massive energy production begins whether we're being chased by a saber-toothed tiger or yelled at by our boss for a substandard report. Now, instead of running into a cave or up a tree to escape, we retreat behind our desks, computers, and phones. The same responses that occurred in early humans take place today, but in today's world there are often few physical outlets for the overload.

Stress, like everything else, has become more complicated. We have more stress factors than ever before. They may not be life-or-death, chased-by-a-tiger stressors; they are often much more subtle. Even a century ago, it might take weeks or even months to get news from another part of the country, and longer from another part of the world. Today we have not only private life and work-related stressors assaulting us, but global worries too. Now we worry not only about our own survival and the survival of our families, but about the survival of the planet. We worry about the destruction of the rain forest. We worry about pornography on the Internet. We read the paper and hear about murders, rapes, and robberies that take place in our own neighborhoods and on the other side of the world.

To add to all of this, we have an array of unhealthy stimulants available to us, from coffee, cigarettes, and legal and illegal drugs, to alcohol, sugar, and refined and processed foods.

How to cope with all this stress? Many of us, especially fast burners, move into a high state of alarm and stay there for long periods of time. Think of your body as a manual car. When you're in first gear, the engine is flooded with a burst of fuel so that you can go from zero to twenty and get the car moving. Then you shift into second gear, which decreases the flow of fuel but keeps the engine running at a steadier pace. As you increase your speed even more, you shift again to keep the flow of fuel consistent with the speed of the car.

When you're stuck in the state of alarm, it's as if you are driving your car from zero to sixty with no shifting whatsoever. There's an enormous infusion of stress hormones overwhelming your body. You're stuck in first gear throughout. You wake up, have your coffee, shovel in some carbohydrates, have some more coffee; when you get to work, you continue to fuel yourself with coffee and carbohydrates all day. You're in an atmosphere that stimulates stress from nine to five (and maybe longer). You're living in an artificially constructed environment where you're "fighting" or "fleeing" all day long.

What happens then is that we go directly from alarm to exhaustion, without passing go and without collecting £200. We burn out, and even though we may continue to function, we do so at greatly reduced capacities.

STRESS AND FOOD

Stress and burnout can occur in so many circumstances that they often take us by surprise. We think we can handle ourselves and adapt to changing situations, and in most ways, we do. But for many of us, the first thing to go in a stressful situation is our relationship with food.

> Susannah came to me at the end of her first year at university. She was feeling sluggish and overweight and wanted to regain her health before the new term began in the autumn. She did well on the Balance program all through the summer. She lost weight, she had more energy, and she was feeling good about herself.

> Then she started classes again, and I didn't see her for about a month and a half. When she returned to my office, she didn't look well. She had gained weight, and her fatigue had returned. I asked her what happened. "The new term started," she said. She had early classes that went for long periods of time. She was eating in the canteen. She had evening classes or would study at the library until late in the evening. It was a more difficult term than she had anticipated, and the easiest way to deal with the stress was to go back to old eating habits of grabbing whatever was available during the day and getting a Chinese take-away every night. She couldn't even think of what her other options might be.

> It wasn't until we sat down and went over her schedule that she realized she could prepare foods the night before to take

The Balance

with her to class as snacks during breaks, that she could bring her lunch in her rucksack or have a salad in the canteen and make healthy choices. We mapped out a time for her to go food shopping once a week so that she'd have a fully stocked refrigerator and cupboard.

A month later, she returned to see me again. She had dropped a substantial amount of weight, and her energy was back up to its higher level. She realized that instead of dealing with the stress of the new term, she had found it easier to fall into the typical student's lifestyle. She had compounded the physical and mental stress of the life of a student by adding on the stress caused by eating all the wrong things. When she went back on the program that was right for her, she reduced her stress level tremendously.

We all know that stress influences the way we eat. What we don't always think about is that food influences the stress we have. When fast burners encounter stress, they also often encounter increased appetite. They feel the need to eat almost continually. They often suffer from hyperglycemia, or high blood sugar. Their cortisol levels are high. Essentially, the body is accessing and burning the fuel available in the food that's being eaten, rather than properly accessing stored fat. Therefore, fast burners try to keep themselves going and keep their energy up by eating more sugar and carbohydrates.

Slow oxidizers under stress may not eat as often as fast burners, but they tend to eat fuller meals. Under stress, their thyroid and adrenal glands become sluggish. This results in the slowing down of metabolic activity. Slow burners may spend a lot of time looking for stimulants like sugar and caffeine to keep themselves going.

In either case, the stress and the stress-based eating cause disturbances in a hormone called cholecystokinin (CCK), the substance that triggers satiety (the feeling of being full). CCK signals the brain to say "stop eating." One of the reasons for these disturbances is that, especially when we're under stress, we don't give the hormone time to do its job. We're a country of fast eaters. Fast food is not limited to what is sold at McDonald's or Burger King. Everything becomes fast food. The average person consumes a meal in about eight minutes! That's average—you may be faster.

Think about lunchtime for office workers. In the circumscribed hour we have, we usually spend half of it running errands. Then we have to buy our food and consume it before it's time to head back to work. Or we run down to the sandwich shop; grab a quick sandwich, some crisps, and a soft drink; and take it all back to the desk and eat while we work. A 1997 study conducted by the KFC restaurant chain concluded that more than 55 percent of workers take 15 minutes or less for lunch and that an astonishing 63 percent skip lunch altogether at least once a week. Job pressures are so intense, and lunchtime is so harried, that we hardly ever give the CCK levels a chance to do their job.

The same thing may occur at dinnertime. Most of us eat lunch around 1:00 P.M. By the time we get home, sometime between 6:00 and 8:00 P.M., we're starving. We're stressed out from how the day has gone. Maybe we have a drink before dinner to calm us down. As soon as the bread basket hits the table, whatever control we may have had is gone. We stuff ourselves full once again. We've gone way past our caloric and nutritional requirements. By the time our CCK has a chance to kick in, we're long past satiated and have moved to being overfull. We've stuffed ourselves with extra fuel, but because we don't need it, it is converted into and stored as fat.

THE STRESS TEST

There are some situations in life that are stress inducers, and there's not much anyone can do about them. Things (both good

The Balance

and bad) happen all the time over which we have no control. On the other hand, there are many stress inducers we can reduce or eliminate from our lives. Answer the questions below to find out what kind of stress inducers are influencing your life.

		YES	NO
1.	I drink two or more cups of coffee a day.	☐	☐
2.	I have trouble sleeping.	☐	☐
3.	I wake up frequently at night to urinate.	☐	☐
4.	I live in a noisy environment.	☐	☐
5.	I get very little exercise each day.	☐	☐
6.	I am an exercise fanatic and must work out several hours a day.	☐	☐
7.	I have trouble expressing my feelings to friends and family.	☐	☐
8.	I have difficulty taking time off to enjoy myself and leave work behind.	☐	☐
9.	I eat meals very quickly—in less than ten minutes.	☐	☐
10.	I smoke cigarettes or cigars.	☐	☐
11.	I have more than one glass of alcohol a day.	☐	☐
12.	I consume chocolate and other sweets on a regular basis (several times a week).	☐	☐
13.	I usually let long periods of time go by between physical checkups.	☐	☐

How many questions did you answer "yes" to? The more times you answered yes, the greater the stress in your life. Following the program cannot help you eliminate all stress factors. For example, it won't stop the noise in your environment. But it can help eliminate many of the stress factors. For example, when your energy levels are low, exercise is the last thing you want to do. Even though you may intellectually understand its benefits, you may have great difficulty getting yourself started. The Balance program can help you to make a habit of exercise, which is a wonderful stress reducer.

When your metabolism is out of whack, your body is often governed more by your glands than by your brain. According to Hans Selye, "stress stimulates our glands to make hormones which can induce a kind of drunkenness. . . . We are on guard against external toxicants, but hormones are part of our bodies; it takes more wisdom to recognize and overcome the foe which fights from within." The program can repair this "drunken" imbalance, restore your energy level, and allow you to enjoy the many health benefits of an appropriate nutritional and exercise program.

WAKE UP AND DON'T SMELL THE COFFEE

The Balance is more than a nutritional program. It is designed to improve your overall emotional and physical well-being. To that end, it is important to identify the stressors in your life and to begin to reduce, if not eliminate, them. It is difficult to achieve metabolic balance when your body's systems are being continually thrown off by unhealthy stimulants and toxins. Once you eliminate these substances, you have a clean slate against which to evaluate your basic metabolic health.

Look at your score on the stress test again. Did you answer "yes" to the questions about coffee, cigarettes, alcohol, and sweets? If so, you are, as they say, adding insult to injury. The Balance program does not advocate extremes. I am not going to tell you never to have another glass of wine with dinner or cappuccino with dessert. But it's important to understand that the overuse of these substances is toxic and causes a great amount of stress to the body's hormonal systems.

I intend no offense to Starbuck's coffee chain, but one of the best ways to get started on the Balance program is to get rid of coffee. Coffee isn't the only bad guy as far as stimulants go, but it's the one we turn to most often for that extra burst of energy we think we need. Many people feel that they can't get started in the morning without their coffee fix.

Coffee contains caffeine, which adversely affects the nervous system, including the brain. It increases the blood pressure and also increases the acidity in the stomach, which ultimately causes greater hunger. Too much caffeine brings on a condition called "caffeine nerves," which can manifest itself as anxiety, irritability, lightheadedness, panic attacks, diarrhea, and insomnia. Coffee may exacerbate fibrocystic breast disease in women, and it may prevent iron from being properly used by the body. When you drink as little as two or three cups a day, you can develop caffeine dependency, which means you need your caffeine fix to feel normal. When you stop drinking coffee, you may experience a runny nose, shaky hands, nausea, and even vomiting—symptoms that are also associated with kicking addictions to substances such as cocaine and heroin.

One of the first things I recommend to my clients is that they give up coffee. Whether you're a fast or slow oxidizer, the elimination of this substance will produce enormous physiological relief; in other words, you'll feel much better.

Make a commitment to go without coffee for ninety days. That means stopping all coffee, including decaffeinated. If you can't go cold turkey, try drinking decaf for the first few weeks and then weaning yourself off that. You may find that you need a little bit more sleep than usual. You may experience some headaches, a decrease in energy, and an increase in irritability. In the beginning, take an aspirin or Panadol or Anadin Extra tablet whenever you feel these withdrawal symptoms coming on. (Panadol and Anadin Extra contain a small amount of caffeine and seem to cushion the withdrawal symptoms for some people.) After one or two weeks, you should be able to eliminate those drugs as well.

Another way to deal with the stress of everyday life is to consume alcohol. I have nothing against an occasional glass of wine with dinner or a relaxing drink at a party. Ask yourself, however, if you're using alcohol simply to relax or as a means of avoiding pressures and responsibilities. Unfortunately, alcohol does not relieve stress; it only adds to it. It dehydrates the body. It also contains simple sugars that are easily converted into body fat.

As you continue with the Balance program, you'll find that your desire for these substances will dissolve. Your energy will return to its natural levels. Many of the stress-related diseases you are experiencing will decrease in severity if not disappear altogether. But you cannot achieve The Balance with layers of added stressors inhibiting your body's efficient use of nutrients. Any kind of stress causes chemical reactions that affect your hormones. When the chemical reactions of stress meet up with the chemical reactions of added stressors like caffeine and alcohol, they amplify any problems that already exist.

You don't have to change your eating habits or lifestyle 100 percent, but the more you can relieve your body of unnecessary layers of stress, the easier it will be to achieve The Balance.

5

EATING LIKE CRAZY

STILL CRAZY AFTER ALL THESE YEARS

This chapter is about things that make you crazy. Crazy in terms of being manic, moody, irritable, addicted, anxious, and depressed. It's about how sugar makes you crazy and how certain other carbohydrates make you crazy. It's about free radicals, what they are, and how they make you crazy. Why you binge and fast and how that makes you crazy. It's about all the things we do to ourselves in the name of food and why we feel bad so much of the time.

If you've been in therapy for five or ten years and you're not much better now than you were when you started, could it possibly be that the food you're eating is contributing to your state of mind? You bet it could. If you start out the day overloaded with anxiety, it could be that the caffeine you're ingesting is wreaking havoc with your nervous system. And if you, like the average American, consume more than 130 pounds of sugar each year, could that possibly be a factor in your inexplicable mood swings? No doubt about it!

If someone were giving you amphetamines and depressants all day long, every day—making you alternately hyperactive and exhausted—you'd know that it was the drugs that were affecting you and not something innately wrong with you. You'd know that you weren't really crazy, that drugs were causing the hills and valleys you laboriously traveled every day. Yet we drug ourselves constantly, repeatedly traversing those hills and valleys, blaming our lack of energy on the fact that we're lazy and blaming our overindulgence in snacks and sweets on the lack of will power. We drug ourselves with food every day without being consciously aware of what we're doing. Then we wonder why things are so out of control and why our lives are so insane.

The purpose of this chapter is to let you know that you are not crazy. It may be that the foods you are eating, just like certain drugs (including medications), are altering your consciousness and affecting your emotional well-being. This chapter will help you understand that in achieving The Balance, you will learn to choose foods that do not make you crazy, foods that will make you feel balanced, controlled, and robust. The Balance is designed to give you the healthy, productive life you were born to have.

GROWING UP SUGAR-FROSTED AND CANDY-COATED

I was raised on a typical American diet, as were most people I know. I was a real sugar baby. I'd get up in the morning and have a big glass of juice along with a bowl of some kind of sugar-frosted cereal with milk. Most of the time, I'd add another teaspoon or two of sugar myself just to be sure it was sweet enough.

Lunches at school consisted of a couple of slices of white bread with margarine, maybe a bowl of soup, a couple of frankfurters, some crisps, and a jelly dessert. Dinner at home could be anything from hamburgers and chips to steak and white rice, with canned or frozen vegetables. There was always bread and butter on the table.

And then there were sweets. I loved sweets. I don't remember any time in my childhood when I didn't have a chocolate bar in my mouth. I was addicted to fizzy drinks at an early age. There was always some in the fridge, and I drank it all day long, whenever I could. By the time I was in my early twenties, I gave up some of the fizzy drinks and started drinking four to five cups of coffee a day. Breakfast then was usually a muffin (maybe two) with a cup of coffee (maybe two). Lunch would be a tuna sandwich, a gherkin, and two Cokes. A Danish and a cup of coffee (maybe two) were my choices for a midday pick-me-up. Dinner was typically chicken, an iceberg lettuce salad, mashed potatoes with butter, and a big bowl of ice cream for pudding. When I put all this down on paper, it seems that it must be exaggerated, but that was how I ate then and how many people eat today.

I paid for my terrible eating habits. At the age of twenty-four, I had already had two teeth removed and well over thirty cavities. I had bleeding gums. I was tired all the time. I was especially vulnerable to the flu and colds. Most people get two or three colds a year, but I got four or five. When I was young, my parents kept me home from school a lot, especially when the colds began to develop into earaches and ear infections.

Then, of course, there were the migraine headaches, which led me into the field of nutrition. My mother has suffered from them all her life, and when I began to get them in my early twenties, I saw the same fate in store for me. When the medical doctors couldn't find anything wrong with me and told me there was nothing they could do, I began making changes in my life. I changed my lifestyle. I put out the cigarettes, put down the fizzy drink bottles, and put away my coffee cup. I slowly became aware that the way I had been eating all my life was killing me.

As we come to a greater understanding of the connection between food and health, we come to the inevitable conclusion that there is a direct relationship between what we eat and what we are. There's no escaping the fact that our tissue is made up of what we consume on a regular basis. It's simple. When we eat foods with health benefits for our specific type (as outlined in chapters 8, 9, and 10), our body remains in good health. When we constantly eat foods that are not only unhealthy but are downright dangerous, our health deteriorates. While we're spending time looking for the magic pill that can make us thin and give us long lives, we overlook the very substances that are available to us every day: lean proteins; fresh fruits and vegetables; and complex, fiber-filled carbohydrates.

THE SUGAR BLUES

We can't blame everything on sugar. Sugar is not the root of all nutritional evil. But the *overconsumption* of sugar is epidemic in America and Britain, where millions of people are experiencing serious sugar addictions, which are leading to serious health problems. Dr. Jacqueline Krohn wrote in her book, *The Whole Way to Allergy Relief and Prevention*, that "sugar depletes the body of specific nutrients including B complex vitamins, magnesium, chromium and other minerals. Ingested sugar destroys the germ killing capacities of the white blood cells for approximately four hours." When the immune system, the body's defense mechanism against disease, is depleted by the ingestion of sugar, the time is ripe for illness to strike.

In chapter 3, I explained that the human body has been genetically and evolutionarily designed to crave sweets because it doesn't manufacture vitamin C. The craving for sweets solved

The Balance

a number of problems for the evolving *Homo sapiens*. As we hunted and gathered our food, we could pick berries and other fruit, which, in their whole form, gave us quick fuel, the vitamin C we needed, and the added benefit of the fibers that are present in fruit. Our sweet tooth was critical in guiding us toward the foods that were nutritionally good for us.

If you follow that sweet tooth forward many thousands of years, into the modern supermarket, you see that we now drink fruit juice, from which we get the sugar but not the fiber. You see that since sweets are available to us in hundreds of forms, there is practically no restraint on the number of things we can buy to satisfy that craving. This has made many of us sugarholics and has set the scene for how poorly we feel. There's only so much sugar our bodies can take in before metabolic disturbances occur.

In his famous 1975 book *Sugar Blues*, William Dufty explained that for the body, particularly the brain, to run at its most efficient level, the amount of glucose (digested sugar) in the blood must balance with the amount of oxygen. When we ingest too much sugar, the body goes into a crisis mode.

When sugar comes into the body, insulin is released from the pancreas. Its job is to escort glucose into the cells, where it can be "burned," used as fuel for energy. Usually only a small amount of insulin is needed to do the job. Under normal circumstances, sugar levels increase and decrease all the time, as both insulin and glucose do their jobs. It's like the gentle wave action found in a lake.

But when we eat a sugar-loaded meal or snack (which includes highly processed carbohydrates as well, since they also are broken down into glucose almost immediately), the gentle lake turns into an ocean tidal wave. The pancreas, alerted to the sudden sugar overload, overreacts and produces large amounts of insulin. We end up with that familiar sudden burst of energy, which makes us feel "up" and energized, followed by a just as sudden descent, when the bottom drops out and we're so tired we can't keep our eyes open. Then, to get through the rest of the day, we grab for a quick fix—a chocolate bar, a bag of crisps—for another energy burst.

The effects of this continual up-and-down pattern can be truly detrimental. As William Dufty put it in *Sugar Blues*, "the end result is damaged adrenals. They are worn out not from overwork but from continual whiplash. Overall production of hormones is low.... Day-to-day efficiency lags, we're always tired, never seem to get anything done. We've really got the sugar blues."

INSULIN RESISTANCE AND THE BALANCE

When the cells are subjected to sugar overload time and time again, the sensors that are normally receptive to insulin begin to shut down. When that happens, a condition called *insulin resistance* develops. In order to compensate for the reduction in receptivity to insulin, the body begins producing larger and larger amounts. This in turn causes increases in appetite and in the conversion of sugar to fat. Not everyone who is a sugarholic develops insulin resistance; it is probably caused by both overindulgence and genetic factors. But the genetic factors alone are not enough to cause the problem. The trouble begins when the sugar intake is higher than normal over a long period of time.

Often when insulin levels are high, blood sugar levels are low; the condition is called *hypoglycemia*. When insulin resistance occurs, insulin levels are high, but so are blood sugar levels because the cells are no longer responding to insulin. When the insulin levels are severely elevated and there's too much insulin in the blood, the condition is called *hyperinsulinemia*. This in turn can lead to such problems as obesity, high blood pressure, high cholesterol, heart disease, and diabetes.

There is no known cure for insulin resistance, but there is a drug-free way to keep your hormones regulated, and that is by controlling what you put in your mouth. All those doughnuts, chocolate bars, fizzy drinks, cakes, pastries, and ice cream are not only making you fat, they're also creating a serious imbalance in your hormonal systems. Food is a drug, and it can manipulate hormone levels. The right foods can stabilize your blood sugar and insulin levels so that the tidal wave effect is calmed down to the gentle waves that keep you functioning at your highest levels.

When you eat the right foods, the ones that are best for your specific metabolic type, you are keeping your hormones working at peak efficiency. Your insulin and glucose levels will rebalance. Read (or reread) chapter 8 if you're a slow burner, chapter 9 if you're a fast burner, and chapter 10 if you're a mixed burner. Whichever type you are, you need to substitute the overconsumption of refined carbohydrates and sugars with greater consumption of high-quality lean proteins such as fish and seafood. You need to add fiber-rich vegetables like broccoli, cabbage, squash, peppers, green beans, and asparagus. And you need to consume more complex carbohydrates like sweet potatoes, squash, and brown rice.

SUGAR AND THE BRAIN: WHY JOHNNY CAN'T THINK STRAIGHT

When you eat the healthy food described in the preceding paragraph, your body—and your mind—can function at peak efficiency. But what happens when you don't maintain a healthy lifestyle? When you continually feed your precious organs with junk food and empty calories? Efficiency turns to deficiency, and peak performance turns to barely getting by.

Your brain is the most important organ you have; it controls all the other organs. It controls your movements, thoughts, and moods, and it regulates your breathing, heartbeat, and body temperature. We're all concerned about what unhealthy eating does to our heart, liver, and kidneys, but we hardly ever think about what this kind of diet is doing to the brain. The brain is often the most poorly nourished organ in the human body.

Your brain, weighing in at about three pounds (nearly 1½ kilograms), constitutes about 2 percent of your total body weight, yet it uses 20 percent of the body's total energy supply. The brain is an energy hog. It needs large amounts of fuel in the form of the chemical adenosine triphosphate (ATP). All the other organs in the body have a choice; they can burn either fat or sugar as fuel. But the brain has no choice. It can burn only sugar as fuel (unless it's literally starving).

Because sugar can't be stored away like fat, the brain depends on a continuous supply of sugar from the bloodstream. In fact, the brain uses about 50 percent of all the sugar in the blood. So what happens when there's a sugar overload and the body reacts by overproducing insulin—the hormone that reduces the amount of blood sugar? According to James South, director of research at Source Naturals and author of *Optimal Nutrition Review*, "when there is little or no insulin in the bloodstream, most organs and tissues . . . will ignore sugar passing through them. Instead, they will burn fat as their energy fuel . . . thereby leaving most of the blood sugar for the brain."

When the sugar overload increases the amount of insulin in the body, all the organs in the body, including the heart, liver, lungs, and muscles, begin to take in sugar from the blood, leaving less of it available to the brain. Although it seems that sugar will provide the quick energy fix we're looking for, the opposite is true. Sugar triggers excessive insulin release, and it reduces the amount of fuel the brain needs to function most efficiently. According to South, complex carbohydrate foods, such as whole grains, vegetables, beans and peas, and nuts and seeds, are a much better source for extra energy because they "require a much longer digestion time than simple sugar foods, so the sugar they produce will trickle into the bloodstream slowly. This provides a much gentler rise in the blood sugar, avoiding the necessity for the brain to trigger an insulin blast, which in turn will leave the brain free to grab all the sugar it needs, without competition from the rest of the body."

THE MOODY BLUES

When the brain is undernourished, it's not just our physical health that suffers. Our state of mind is affected as well. Although we may not always be aware of it, we frequently use food as a mood-altering drug. Those ups and downs of energy caused by too much sugar and refined carbohydrates also cause us to alternate between depression and euphoria. When we get that sugar high, we're ready for anything. Then, as blood sugar levels dissipate, we begin to feel worse and worse. To varying degrees, we get irritable, shaky, nervous, or depressed. So we begin to eat like crazy again, gobbling down more sugar and carbohydrates. In extremes of anxiety and depression, we may resort to binge eating in an overzealous attempt to modulate our moods.

This behavior has its consequences. The overconsumption of carbohydrates and sweets may produce some instant gratification, a druglike high, but it is transitory. The effect will pass soon enough, but not before it has stripped away and cannibalized essential nutrients the body requires. When the high passes, it leaves us weaker, duller, and for those who are predisposed to gain weight, always a little bit heavier than we were before.

What causes these changes in mood chemistry? Recently, scientists have been pointing more and more toward a brain chemical called *serotonin*. Serotonin is a neurotransmitter that helps send messages across synapses (gaps between nerve cells) in the brain. It seems that serotonin plays a central role in mood and emotion. Some neurotransmitters carry messages about what's happening around us—the temperature, the sounds we hear, the things we see—and translate them into useful information. Other neurotransmitters lead us to action, telling the muscles what to do. However, serotonin works on a more emotional level. As Michael Lemonick wrote in a *Time* magazine article in September of 1997, "other neurotransmitters help us know when our stomachs are full; serotonin tells us whether we feel satisfied." Other chemicals help us perceive the water level in a glass; serotonin helps us decide whether we will think of it as half empty or half full.

Low levels of serotonin have been linked to such conditions as depression, overeating, bulimia, obsessive-compulsive disorder, autism, PMS, migraine headaches, schizophrenia, and even violent and criminal behavior.

High serotonin levels make us feel relaxed and more in control. It seems that when serotonin levels are optimum, we are better able to resist temptation and are able to function on a fairly even keel without wildly fluctuating mood swings. Popular antidepressant drugs such as Elavil and Prozac work because they affect serotonin levels. Such drugs have also been used as treatment for weight control, but recent events concerning Redux (dexfenfluramine) and fenfluramine have shown that we have a lot to learn about both the brain and drugs of this kind before they can become a healthy solution for weight reduction.

These diet drugs were designed to stimulate nerve endings to release extra serotonin into nerve synapses. But what the drug companies did not discover in time was that the use of Redux and fenfluramine (as well as phentermine, a drug that is related to fenfluramine and was prescribed together with it in a combination popularly called fen/phen) could result in abnormalities in the shape of the heart valves, an extremely serious and potentially fatal condition. In September of 1997, just a year and a half after they were introduced, these drugs were pulled off the market.

We don't need drugs to regulate the level of serotonin. It can be done with food every day. When we consume carbohydrates, our serotonin level goes up. We eat to make ourselves feel better. And it works—for a while. As we're eating these carbohydrates, however, we're also getting fatter, and the heavier we are, the more serotonin it takes to elevate our mood. It's just like the tolerance we build up for almost every drug we take: The more of it we use, the more we need to get the same effect.

Clearly, many factors contribute to our state of mind. The brain is so complex it would be impossible and irrational to say that only by eating the right foods can we cure depression, anxiety, and other emotional problems. We all have life issues to deal with; we're all contending with a myriad of problems on a regular basis. We have economic problems, environmental problems, and relationship problems. Neither drugs nor healthy eating can eliminate these problems, but dealing with them can be made easier.

Many of my clients who are in therapy report that their therapy sessions are much more productive when they follow the guidelines of the Balance program. They are able to think more clearly and have more energy to take actions to solve their problems. It doesn't seem to be enough to try to understand who we are in light of our personal histories and our upbringing. To get a complete picture, we have to inject our dietary history as well. To a large extent, we are what we have consumed.

FREE RADICALS AND WHY
THEY MAKE US CRAZY

It's important, in terms of understanding how our diets are killing us, to take into consideration the role of free radicals. A free radical is an oxygen molecule with an odd number of electrons in the outer ring of one of its atoms. Free radicals are unstable because of their missing electrons. To try to correct this condition, free radicals grab onto healthy cells and try to "steal" their electrons. What results, however, is that more free radicals are created, causing a chain reaction. Free radicals have the potential to create a tremendous amount of cellular damage.

There are many different kinds of cells in the body. Some, such those in the skin, the lining of the intestinal tract, and the blood, are continuously worn out and have the ability to replace themselves. Other tissues, such as those in the brain, nerves, and muscles (including the heart), cannot replace themselves once they are worn out. Cell membranes are destroyed. Essential enzymes are damaged. Nutrients can't reach cell membranes. Genes and chromosomes mutate. Over time, free radical activity can produce extremely damaged and, in some instances, malignant cells.

Where do free radicals come from? Free radicals are continuously produced as a natural result of many of the body's essential chemical reactions. Free radicals are produced naturally as oxygen interacts with organic matter. If you take an apple, cut into it, and leave it out on your counter, it begins to turn brown. As it interacts with oxygen in the air, it oxidizes, which means it is succumbing to free radical damage. If you leave any kind of food out on the counter, it will begin to spoil from contact with free radicals in the air.

If you leave a bicycle outside and allow it to interact with the elements, sooner or later it, too, will begin to oxidize. It begins to rust away. You and I are in large measure rusting away as well.

We are oxidizing. We are succumbing to the effects of free radical activity. However, we can increase or decrease the rate at which we're "spoiling" by what we consume.

What happens to food when we refine it? We increase its free radical potential. Oils, for instance, are easily radicalized. Free radical damage increases in fats and in oils much more so than in any other substances. When we superheat an oil and then fry food in it, we exponentially increase the free radical volume of both the oil and the food that's being fried. When we eat that food, we ingest extremely high amounts of free radicals. Chips, white bread, fried chicken, and most fast foods all contain high levels of free radicals.

All of these foods that are high in fat and in free radicals contribute to the free radical buildup in our bodies. Our bodies are designed to deal with only so much free radical exposure on a daily basis. Once we go past that free radical threshold, the free radical waste begins to age our cells prematurely. It contributes to the degenerative diseases of the modern world and can lead to an early demise.

ANTIOXIDANTS TO THE RESCUE

We are predisposed to diseases like arthritis, chronic fatigue syndrome, hormonal imbalances in women, diabetes, and cancer by an inherent dysfunction of our genes. Scientists are constantly discovering gene mutations that make us predisposed to these illnesses. Not everyone who has these gene mutations becomes ill, however. It may be possible to stave off the inherited tendencies by changing our diet. If a gene that is already weak is attacked by a free radical, disastrous results can occur. That is why the introduction of antioxidants into the diet is so important.

The reason that foods have preservatives added to them is to slow down the effects of oxidation. If you go to the supermarket and read the labels, you'll see many packaged foods with long list of added preservatives. Those preservatives are added to slow down the oxidation process. The manufacturer has added antioxidants intended to reduce free radical activity so the food will last longer on the shelf.

Introducing antioxidants into our bodies will slow down the degenerative process. We do this, not with the chemicals food manufacturers use, but with the diet and supplements of the Balance program. Supplements such as vitamin C, vitamin E, and beta-carotene are effective antioxidants. In fact, recent studies have shown that the consumption of vitamin E can offset the advance of Alzheimer's disease by up to a year.

There are also foods that are natural antioxidants. Cruciferous vegetables like broccoli, cauliflower, cabbage, and kale all have natural anticancer properties. They're high in naturally occurring antioxidants. So are foods high in beta-carotene, such as carrots, tomatoes, courgettes, and squash. Root vegetables are also high in antioxidants. Try adding parsnips and sweet potatoes to your diet, as well as spinach and brussels sprouts. Foods that are highest in vitamin C include green peppers, broccoli, brussels sprouts, cauliflower, strawberries, spinach, oranges, grapefruit, and carrots.

THE THERAPEUTIC EFFECTS OF THE BALANCE

Throughout the last four chapters, we've shown that modern society suffers from a kind of nutritional schizophrenia. We are concerned with nutrition, but we want our treats at the same time. We have so much stress and so little time, we often eat too fast and too much. We *think* we don't have time for nutrition. In fact, our interest in nutrition is on the decline. In a survey conducted by Yankelovich Partners, a Connecticut-based research and consulting company, twenty-five hundred Americans were asked whether they paid as much attention to nutrition when they ate out as when they ate at home. In 1994, 40 percent answered yes. In 1997, only 36 percent gave the same response. In 1995, 37 percent of respondents said that weight concerned them. In 1997, that number had dropped to only 29 percent.

As a nation, we are eating ourselves crazy and out of control. The Balance is a way to regain that control. It's about a way of life that helps us to remain sane. Unfortunately, we love the foods that make us crazy. Who doesn't love ice cream dripping in chocolate fudge sauce, scones with clotted cream and jam or a big bag of chips? These are foods that we don't want to give up. The Balance doesn't require you to be perfect. If you want to indulge once in a while, no major harm will be done.

If you constantly indulge in these kinds of foods, however, tremendous harm will be done. The result will be premature aging of the heart and brain, not to mention the teeth, skin, and hair. Gradually replacing the foods that make you crazy with the foods that make you healthy is what The Balance is all about. The programs outlined in chapters 8, 9, and 10 will restore balance and sanity in your life, and help make you strong and lean. How you feel when you wake up in the morning can be directly traced back to what you ate the night before. This is what you need to remember as you construct a new way of eating that doesn't make you crazy.

6

WOMEN AND WEIGHT: WINNING THE LOSING BATTLE

THE SAD STATISTICS

In 1997, *Psychology Today* magazine polled 3,452 women about their body image. Fifteen percent said they would sacrifice more than five years of their lives to be the weight they wanted. Twenty-four percent said they would give up more than three years.

In a 1995 *Life* magazine article, a member of Overeaters Anonymous, when warned that her eating disorder could kill her, was quoted as saying, "As long as I'm thin in the casket and people walk by and say, 'Oh, my gosh, look how thin she is,' I really wouldn't mind dying on a diet."

Eating disorders are rampant in our society. Conservative estimates suggest that diseases such as anorexia nervosa and bulimia affect 1–2 percent of the female population. In the US, congresswoman Nita Lowey is setting up a federal information and education program about eating disorders. In an article in the November 1997 issue of *Women's News*, she quoted the following statistics: "Although eating disorders are curable, the majority of people afflicted by them suffer for years. Over 31 percent of people with eating disorders have the diseases for 6 to 10 years, and 16 percent have the diseases for 11 to 15 years. Incredibly, 50 percent of those suffering are never cured. . . . Worse, approximately six percent of those with the diseases will die from it."

These are startling and disturbing statistics. You don't have to have a serious eating disorder to suffer the consequences of our society's obsession with women's weight. The 1995 *Life* magazine article cites a study by Dr. Steven L. Gortmaker of the Harvard School of Public Health who conducted an eight-year study of more than ten thousand women. He found that, compared with thinner women, overweight women were 20 percent less likely to get married, earned $6,710 or £10,000 less per year (on average), and were 10 percent more likely to be living below the poverty level.

THE SAD STORIES

What do all these numbers mean? They mean that women, especially overweight women (and women who *think* they are overweight), have a tough time in our society. I first began to realize how serious this problem was in the early 1980s, when two colleagues and I started a program called Women and

Weight (which we later renamed Lighten Up: Food, Weight and Self-Image). We held two-day workshops for about fifty women at a time. The women were of all ages, economic groups, and ethnic backgrounds. Some were thin, some were very heavy; all had problems with food.

We did an exercise called the Hot Seat, in which a woman would get up in front of the group and talk about her relationship to and history with food. Extraordinary experiences were shared. One woman, who didn't want her husband to know about her obsession with food and her secret night eating, would cut out the bottom of the ice cream container and push it up toward the top so that if he opened the container, it would appear to be full. A young Jamaican woman told of how her mother and father had locked her in the basement and brought in a *santero* (a Caribbean witch doctor), who sacrificed some birds and a goat to try to get her to stop bingeing and start losing weight. A rail-thin model stood up in front of the room and wept over how fat she considered herself to be.

In fact, it appears that some women see themselves as fat no matter how much they weigh. Scientists have known for many years that women who suffer from anorexia see themselves as overweight despite what the mirror and scales tell them. But a 1986 study by Kevin Thompson reported in *Psychology Today* revealed that more than ninety-five percent of normal-size women he studied overestimated their body sizes as at least one-fourth larger than they actually were.

I am working now with another model who constantly tells me she is bloated and is putting on weight. Yet to look at her, you would think, "How much thinner can she get?" She represents the overall indoctrination of the Western psyche that thin is beautiful, thin is "better." We have begun to deify dieting and weight loss almost as a religion. The pursuit of thinness became the late-twentieth-century equivalent of the pursuit of spirituality.

Go to any newsagent, and the tabloid headlines will scream the news of the latest big star to get even bigger. No matter how juicy the rest of the scandals may be, it seems there is no crime worse than gaining weight. Stars like Elizabeth Taylor, Kirstie Alley, and Alicia Silverstone have all had their bodily ups and downs publicly recorded. In reality, even at their heaviest they are thinner than most of the people reading the magazine, so what does that do to the psyche of the woman standing in front of the cashier bringing home a cartful of goodies for herself and her family?

We live in a culture in which we are, to a large extent, out of touch with what inherently produces happiness. We focus on image and external packaging. We fall for every diet scam that comes along, pursuing fantastic wishful thinking because we think it will make us happy. We follow the religion of weight loss, no matter how ineffective and unsatisfying it turns out to be. We are disappointed over and over again as we focus on how we look and not how we feel. We pursue thinness, not well-being. We've lost the context, and we are stuck in the details. So we return to dieting, even though we know it doesn't work.

HOW IT ALL STARTED

In the early 1800s, being overweight was a sign of prosperity. Only those in the wealthy upper classes could afford to eat well. But by the turn of the century, when agriculture was booming in this country and factory workers in the cities could afford more substantial meals, even the middle class began to put on weight. It then became fashionable for the upper classes to slim down.

By 1901, insurance companies began to stress the link between overweight and early death. However, as Laura Fraser says in her excellent book *Losing It: America's Obsession with Weight and the Industry That Feeds on It*, "none of the early insurance charts was based on data about women; the conclusions about women were made up from data about a rather narrow population group, men who were old and wealthy enough to get life insurance."

In the 1920s, the fashionable flappers marked the beginning of the idealization of the thin, flat-chested look. Clothes were now being mass produced rather than tailor-made to hide any figure flaws. Penny scales popped up everywhere, and the diet industry was on its way. Some psychologists, including Dr. Brett Silverstein of New York's City College, who has studied women's fashions throughout the twentieth century, suggested that women become thinner and subconsciously adopt a more masculine look when they make the greatest political strides. For example, in the 1920s they had just gained the right to vote, and in the 1960s (remember Twiggy?), feminism began to make great strides. In the 1980s and 1990s, the "dress for success" idea took hold, with many women opting for man-tailored suits (which fit women well only if they have no hips and no bustline) and toned-down business attire.

The obsession with being thin continues today, with even more pressure. The ideal woman now is not only thin, she's superfit and athletic, exercising in the gym or running several miles a day in her "spare time." If you look in the personal ads in any newspaper in any Western city, the two words you will see used over and over by men who are looking for partners are "slim" and "fit." If your body does not qualify in either or both of these categories, don't apply.

Being overweight is not only a handicap in finding a mate. A heavy woman I know (whose husband is also overweight) recently applied to a well-known and highly regarded adoption agency. The couple was turned down because, as they were told straight to their faces, "no birth mother would choose you as potential parents because you are too fat."

No wonder the Centers for Disease Control report that nearly half of all American women are on diets. No wonder being overweight often leads to depression. How can you help but be depressed when your diet works for a short period of time, then lets you down again? When you're walking around hungry all the time, consumed with thoughts about food, waiting for the time when the diet will be over, when you can eat again? When you gain back the weight you lost and more?

Women have an added factor in the fight against being overweight. The woman is usually in charge of the food for her family. Not only is she obsessed with her own food, but she's got to shop and cook to please the other members of her family as well. When she's on a diet, she's often cooking one meal for herself and another meal for the rest of the crew, a situation that only increases the feelings of being left out and deprived.

FATTENING THE DIET INDUSTRY'S COFFERS

It has been estimated that in America alone between $34 and $50 billion is spent every year on dieting. Clearly, the diet industry has a high stake in keeping its customers coming back for more. All kinds of scams have been perpetrated on the public in the name of losing weight. There are creams that will allegedly make our thighs thin, pills that will absorb all the fat before it can be digested, thereby allowing us to eat anything in any amount we wish. In the 1950s, there was a hormone derived from the urine of pregnant women that was supposed to make us thin. There were liquid diets that killed almost sixty people. There is ephedrine (an amphetamine-like substance that is found in many herbal diet remedies) that has caused more than two dozen heart failure deaths and hundreds of close calls. And there are, of course, several prescription drugs that are no less harmful and no more effective than any of the aforementioned products.

Then there are the giant food companies who are working around the clock to develop the latest "diet" products. Procter & Gamble hoped that its fat substitute, olestra, would be a big moneymaker, despite the fact that many consumers complained of a nasty aftertaste, flatulence, and diarrhea. So far, the product has not fulfilled the manufacturer's expectations—only because it doesn't taste that good. It appears that people will eat almost anything as long as it tastes good. In November of 1997, the *New York Times* reported that in a survey conducted by NPD, an Illinois food research company, consumers for the past 17 years were asked whether they agree with the following statement: "The most important thing about food is that it look good, taste good and smell good." For ten years, from 1985 to 1995, 36 percent of respondents said that they agreed with that statement. In 1996, the figure went up to 39 percent, and in 1997, it rose to 40 percent.

Olestra, like thousands of other products, was developed as part of the fat-free food craze. The public has been inundated with appeals to cut out the fat. We have rushed to the supermarket and scoured the shelves looking for foods labeled no fat or low fat. What most of us don't realize is that fat-free products often contain virtually the same number of calories as the fat-filled versions! Fat-free does not mean sugar-free. Equally important, fat-free does not mean calorie-free. In fact, the fat in many of these products is replaced by sugar to maintain the taste. People are consuming whole boxes of fat-free biscuits; filling themselves up with non-nutritive, highly processed carbohydrates; driving blood sugar and insulin levels higher and higher; and setting the stage for fat storage—all the while thinking they are eating in a healthier manner and wondering why they can't seem to lose weight.

People believe what they want to believe. They want to believe there is going to be a biscuit they can eat without consequence. A few years ago, the television program *Remington Steele* featured an episode in which someone had invented a delicious calorie-free chocolate chip cookie. The trouble was, every time someone got hold of the recipe, he or she was found murdered, because whoever was left in possession of that recipe would, of course, be a billionaire. If someone really did invent such a biscuit, he would be king of the world. In our society of wanting it all, calorie-free chocolate chip cookies are high on the list.

ALL FAT IS *NOT* CREATED EQUAL

Weight loss clubs often advise women to use the buddy system—to go on a diet with a friend or spouse as support and encouragement. But if a woman chooses a male partner, she is likely to suffer discouragement instead, because men and women store, use, and lose fat differently. Both genders, however, have certain things in common with other mammals. Studies have shown that all mammals have fat deposits in similar locations around the body.

A 1990 *New York Times* article by Natalie Angier entitled "Fat on Thighs and Paunches Is the Fate of All Mammals" states that "all fat is not created equal. . . . Fat deposits have very different functions, depending on sex and storage sites." It seems that men generally store more of their fat in the abdominal area, and abdominal fat is more responsive to stress hormones. Once again, this seems to be a trait we humans have inherited from our earliest ancestors. Angier quotes Dr. M. C. R. Greenwood, a professor of nutrition at the University of California: "Abdominal fat seems to be a fast-getaway fat store. It's a quickly available energy source for running or fighting or seeking prey. Presumably early man needed to do that, while women needed a long-term energy store for pregnancy and nursing."

Women store more fat in the thighs and buttocks, where it responds to female hormones, providing energy for pregnancy and breast-feeding. Some women, predominantly fast burners, can also develop belly fat. Both men and women who have this apple-shaped body type have a greater risk of cardiovascular problems, such as high blood pressure and heart disease, than do people who have pear-shaped bodies.

Studies have also shown that women have a greater abundance than men of the enzyme lipoprotein lipase (LPL), which helps extract fat from food and store it in fat cells. Not only that, but people who have been overweight for long periods of time tend to have increased levels of LPL, levels that remain high even after weight loss.

This information is included, not to discourage anyone from attempting to lose weight, but to explain why women often have a much more difficult time at it than men do. Women are naturally plumper than men, and there is only so much that can be done to fight mammalian biology.

LEAVING THE NONSENSE BEHIND

How do we get ourselves out from beneath all the pressure to lose weight, all the hype and advertising ballyhoo? It isn't easy. We can't divorce ourselves from the world. A few weeks ago it was Fashion Week in New York, and every night the local news flashed images of "perfect" women strutting down the catwalks, depressing thousands of women in the Greater New York area. These images were followed by commercials for fast-food restaurants, chocolate bars, and frozen pizzas. What's a person to do?

Is it simply a matter of resisting temptation? Of course not. It's a matter of becoming educated. The more you know about how the body functions, about what gives you energy and what makes you fat, the better you will be able to understand what makes you healthy. Only when you have a broad understanding of the interplay between food and your health can you define for yourself the practices and guidelines that will bring you towards a healthier ideal.

The goal of The Balance is not necessarily to lose weight. For most people, that will be a beneficial by-product. This program is designed to make and keep you healthy at a weight that is healthy for you. That weight may be higher than the "ideal" image you're used to seeing in print advertising and on TV. But not everyone is meant to be rail-thin. Each of us has a different weight, or set point, to which we are genetically predisposed. Whether we try to lose past that point, or to gain past that point, the body will struggle to get back to that number.

The Balance allows you to stay comfortably within your natural weight range. It helps you learn to eat in a way that is rational and mature, and that doesn't involve harsh dietary restrictions. This will not only allow you to maintain a fit and healthy body, but will help reduce the risk of illness, especially illnesses that most often affect women.

ISSUES OF WOMEN'S HEALTH

For many years, most of the research that was done in the West about various diseases included only men. It was assumed that what was true for men would be true for women as well. In many instances, that did not turn out to be the case. There are many diseases and disorders that affect predominantly women, including many autoimmune disorders like lupus, chronic fatigue, and osteoporosis. In addition, conditions like PMS and menopause not only are gender-related, but are usually compounded by women's dietary habits and their levels of fitness.

Let's take a look at some of these conditions.

Premenstrual Syndrome

Premenstrual syndrome, more commonly known as PMS, is essentially caused by hormonal imbalances. PMS comes in a variety of forms that have been identified and categorized according to symptoms:

- *PMS type A:* feelings of heightened *a*nxiety and tension
- *PMS type B: b*loating, water retention, breast tenderness
- *PMS type C: c*ravings, mostly for sweets, carbohydrates, and occasionally salt
- *PMS type D: d*epression
- *PMS type E:* a combination of *e*verything in types A through D

Any of these symptoms can be made worse if you are out of balance in diet, exercise, and stress. As the body prepares for menstruation, estrogen levels begin to rise. Estrogen has a high affinity for water; that's one reason you may feel bloated. If you're also eating a lot of salty foods at that time of the month, you're exacerbating the situation.

The hormonal imbalances that occur during PMS can also cause varying degrees of moodiness, anxiety, tension, and depression. Hormones (or lack thereof) affect the way your neurotransmitters function. Many women crave sweets such as chocolates, which are high in magnesium and therefore may have a sedating effect. The chocolate seems to be able to calm those frayed nerves. The problem is that if you become dependent on sweets and other carbohydrates to change your PMS moodiness, it's likely that you'll use them as an ongoing means of dealing with tension and stress throughout the month. In an article titled "Premenstrual Syndrome: A Natural Approach to Management" (*Clinical Nutritional Insights*, July 1997), Dr. Joseph L. Mayo wrote, "Sugar also increases the tendency to hypoglycemia, particularly premenstrually, giving rise to sugar cravings, irritability, and headaches. High sodium intake combined with large intakes of sugar can impact water retention."

A better way of dealing with the physical and psychological discomforts of PMS is to address the hormonal imbalances directly. That means rather than using food as a medication to relieve the symptoms, using food every day to keep the hormones in balance. The foods that are right for your metabolic type will do that.

Stress is another factor that appears to exacerbate premenstrual complaints. Stress can be caused by the typical woman's daily overload of responsibilities, but it can also be caused by stimulants such as alcohol, tobacco, and caffeine. Dr. Mayo wrote, "Caffeine, by increasing the effects of adrenaline, increases the effects of stress and aggravates symptoms such as anxiety, tension, and hypoglycemia. Studies have shown that women who consume large amounts of caffeine are more likely to suffer from PMS."

It has also been scientifically proved that exercise can help reduce stress and thereby reduce the symptoms of PMS. Aerobic conditioning produces endorphins, neurotransmitter-like compounds that work as both a pain reliever and an antidepressant. I suggest to my clients who suffer from PMS that they walk, run, or work out in a health club when symptoms arise.

I also recommend that my clients take supplements (which are considered in depth in chapter 11). One product we have found to provide excellent relief is a combination of herbs, vitamins, and minerals called BioPMT, made by Thorne Research,[1] which you can start taking up to two weeks before you get your period. A combination of supplements found to be effective is as follows:

Magnesium	100 milligrams
Vitamin B6	200 milligrams
Pyridoxal-5-phosphate	50 milligrams
(a complex form of B6)	
Buffered vitamin C	500 milligrams

[1] I have no monetary interest in any of the companies that manufacture or supply the supplements or products I recommend in this book. These products can be found in health food stores.

Another supplement, which I discuss in chapter 11 and list in the glossary, is St. John's wort, which is just starting to become popular in the United States after many years of use in Europe. Taking 300 milligrams after the first meal of the day has been found to be useful in the management of PMS.

THE MENOPAUSE

The menopause happens to every woman, sooner or later. Some women hardly notice the change at all except for the fact that they have stopped menstruating. For others, however, it is an intensely uncomfortable period.

Many people in the modern medical community look at the menopause as another disease that needs to be conquered, rather than as a natural part of a woman's life cycle. The menopause is not a disease, however. It is a disequilibrium that occurs as the body is trying to readjust itself to lower levels of hormones.

Nowadays, women have many options for dealing with this time in their lives. The current medical treatment is hormone replacement therapy (HRT), which has worked well for some women and has caused problems for others. Some women find that they don't do well on hormone replacement therapy because it makes them heavier, hungrier, and more water retentive. Most women have to experiment, and often a combination of traditional medical therapeutics and alternative, or complementary, health practices produces the best results.

One of the most common complaints associated with the menopause is hot flashes. Many women who wake up at night from hot flashes find that they benefit from a combination of the herbs gotu kola and dong quai, which help relieve hot flashes, vaginal dryness, and depression.

Rhonda E. provides a perfect example of the benefits of these herbs. At age forty-nine, she was waking up every night in a pool of sweat. Often, she was so uncomfortable she could not get back to sleep. She was also starting to develop migraine headaches. I put her on a combination of gotu kola and dong quai, and within three days her symptoms had disappeared.

Although I stress the value of eating right for your metabolic type at all times, this is especially important premenstrually and during the menopause. The body is going through many hormonal changes, both major and minor. If your system is out of whack to begin with, influenced by too much sugar and too many carbohydrates, overloaded with caffeine and nicotine, you're going to have a much more difficult time getting relief.

OSTEOPOROSIS

Lately, everyone has been jumping on the calcium bandwagon. Because the body cannot manufacture calcium, we have to get it from outside sources like food and supplements. But like fat, not all calcium is created equal. For instance, there is no reason to take a particular antacid because the advertisements say it contains calcium. Stones that you find on the ground contain calcium, but that doesn't mean your system can break this calcium down, digest it, and use it appropriately for strengthening bones.

I recommend calcium supplements in the form of calcium hydroxyapatite (the most absorbable form of calcium available). A product I recommend that includes calcium in this form is called "For Women Only", manufactured by the Allergy Research Group. Among its other ingredients are an extract of licorice called deglycylrhizinate, the herb dong quai, and vitamin D3. This combination improves the body's use of calcium and stimulates estrogen production.

Exercise is also an important element in preventing osteoporosis. According to Ann Louise Gittleman, in her book *Super Nutrition for Women*, "bones become stronger with physical stress. If they are not used, they lose calcium and become porous. In addition, by strengthening the muscles and tendons that protectively surround bone, exercise makes bones less susceptible to injury." She recommends weight-bearing exercises: "those that cause your muscles to pull on bones to move some or all of your body . . . through space or against gravity," such as walking, jogging, running, and aerobic dancing.

In the next section of the book, I discuss the specifics of the Balance program, including food plans, exercise programs, and supplementation for each metabolic type. The Balance comes from a combination of these three elements. You can't achieve a body in balance by concentrating on one element alone. Eating right for your type is an excellent way to start, but the best way to achieve maximum health is through an individually tailored program of nutritional management, fitness, and cutting edge supplements. The next four chapters show you how to design your own personalized health agenda.

PART II

ACHIEVING BALANCE

7

INTRODUCTION TO GOOD EATING

CHANGING FOR THE BETTER

Earlier in this book, I said that taking the metabolic type test in chapter 2 would change your life. That was a slight exaggeration. Simply taking the test and finding out what type you are won't change your life all by itself. It's what you do with that knowledge that counts.

There may be many reasons to *want* to change your life. You may want to lose weight. You may have a specific illness you want to heal. You may want to lead a more active life, be more productive at work, or simply be a healthier person. These are all worthy goals. Yet most of us run into an all-too-common stumbling block that seems to pervade modern life: We want to change our lives, but we don't want to have to make changes to do it.

It could be that you, like millions of others, are focusing on the wrong end of the stick. You complain about your weight, about your aches and pains, about the fact that you don't feel up to par. Perhaps you feel that you're not getting enough out of life. But do you ever ask yourself, "Am I putting enough in?"

Are you simply waiting to feel better? Waiting until you're on a better financial footing? Until the next project is completed? Until the first of the month, or the first of the year? Have you waited long enough? If you have, you can start making changes right now.

It isn't as though everything is going to change overnight when you start eating right for your metabolic type. In fact, the more gradual the change, the more likely it is to be a permanent one. This is not a quick weight loss program. This is a program geared to giving you antidotes to the conditions in which you find yourself. By following the Balance program, you greatly improve your potential for weight loss. You improve your potential for increasing your energy and productivity, and for extending—and enjoying—your life. Aren't these things worth working for?

The Balance program can give you a new perspective on the "problem" of health and well-being. The concept I'm espousing is pragmatism. To know your metabolic type and eat accordingly is pragmatic. It gives you an advantage. To understand how the hormone systems in your body work, and how various supplements can enhance those systems, is pragmatic. It gives you an advantage. Learning how to exercise in the way that benefits you most is pragmatic, and it gives you an advantage.

That is the whole point. Why not do everything possible to develop the most advantageous way of taking care of yourself?

That may mean making changes, but it doesn't mean you have to change your entire life in one day. It means taking things slowly so that both your mind and your body have time to adapt.

> I worked with Stan L. for six months on changing his breakfast pattern. He was always in such a rush to get to work (and always late), he'd grab a cup of black coffee and a doughnut from the sandwich shop next door to his office and then wonder why he was falling asleep halfway through the morning (which made him grab another cup of coffee). It took him all those months to recognize the advantages of waking up half an hour earlier to eat an appropriate breakfast at home. As he gradually developed that habit, he was able to slow himself down and be less rushed on his way to work every day, and still get there on time. He no longer needed several cups of coffee to keep himself awake in the morning. He worked at a good steady pace until lunchtime. He couldn't believe that these changes would come about just by eating a healthy breakfast, yet this minor change in his lifestyle made a major difference in his life.

LEARN TO WORK WITH WHAT YOU'VE GOT

There is one important point to remember regarding The Balance: It is not "better" to be one metabolic type than another. Being fast, slow, or mixed is simply a category of your oxidation potential, a commentary on your capacity to burn fuel. It's not good or bad to be fast or slow. The idea is not to try to change a slow burner to a fast burner, or vice versa, or to change everyone into a mixed burner. It's more like the U.S. Army slogan: "Be the best that you can be." If you're a slow burner, you don't want to be so slow that it's detrimental to your health. You want to function at optimum slow burner levels. If you're a fast burner, you don't want to be speeding out of control. Again, you want to reach optimum levels. And if you're a mixed burner, you want to stay within a healthy range and not veer off to either extreme.

It is also important to note that persons of any metabolic type can be fit and trim or can have problems with weight. Some people will always be heavier than others. If you have an unrealistic weight goal, you will find yourself constantly frustrated when you are unable to reach it. You cannot change your genetic predisposition. If you are five feet, five inches, for instance, that height was programmed into your genes. There isn't anything you can do about it; it is something you can't change. Your genes have also given you a certain body type. You may never be model-thin. Fortunately, you can do more about your weight (and your entire level of fitness) than you can about your height.

There are three factors that determine your weight and fitness. They are genetics, diet, and exercise. You can't rearrange your genes, but you can change your nutritional habits and you can exercise. You can look at your "weight gene" the same way you look at your "intellect gene." Many people believe that intellect is like a jar. Some people come into the world with a small jar, some with a medium-size jar, and some with a huge jar. Most of us never fill the jar we're given, so how big the jar was to start with may not matter. It is how you fill the jar you are given that is important.

Before you throw in the towel and say, "There's nothing I can do, it's all in my genes," ask yourself if you've done everything in your power to fill the "jar" you have been given. If you have a genetic predisposition to gain weight, are you doing everything you can to counteract that predisposition? Are you making a sincere effort to be healthy? Or are you filling your jar with junk food and a sedentary lifestyle? It may be more difficult for you to lose weight than it is for someone who is genetically predisposed to be thin. Even if you do make significant changes in your diet and exercise program, you may never have the body of a model or a marathoner, but you can certainly have a healthy, fit body.

"TELL ME WHAT TO EAT!"

One of the challenges many people face when they decide they want to have a healthy, fit body is the overwhelming amount of information out there. Deciding which foods to eat can be confusing, to say the least. When clients come into my office for the first time, the most common question they ask is, "What should I eat?" They usually ask this question soon after they take a seat, before I've had a chance to learn anything about them. In that case, it's a difficult question to answer. It all depends on biochemical individuality. There is no perfect diet that applies to everyone.

No food is intrinsically good or bad. Its value depends on how the food affects you. A meal is like the opening night of a show. The audience watches the show, applauds, and thinks, "That was fantastic! Everything was perfect." The ingenue goes home thinking, "What a lemon. I hardly get any time on stage at all." The costume designer, watching the same show, thinks, "The show was not very good. There was a ladder in the star's stocking, and the leading man's trousers were too long!" The musical director thinks, "It was a disaster. The tempo in the first act finale was much too slow!"

In the same way, you might look at a meal and think it is perfect, while your friend turns up her nose and says, "How can you eat that thing?" Although there are guidelines that should be followed, exactly what you eat depends on your personal preferences, your lifestyle, and your food sensitivities. If I recommend that strawberries are a good fruit choice (which I do), and you are allergic to strawberries, I certainly don't expect you to include them in your food plan. If I recommend fish as a good choice of protein (which I do), and you hate fish, I hope that you will make an effort to eat it at least once in a while, but I don't expect you to consume foods you loathe. Don't think you have to abandon healthy eating altogether because you can't or won't eat one recommended element.

We need to evaluate nutritional advice by looking at the available evidence and forming an opinion. Although the field of nutrition is exciting at this time, with new discoveries being made every day, the changes can be confusing. Things that were said to be bad for us yesterday may be deemed tomorrow's panacea. Therefore, it's important that you incorporate your own judgment when looking at all the information that's being presented to you, in this book and in any others you may read.

Fitness expert Jonathan Bowden, director of the Equinox Training Institute (part of the Equinox Fitness clubs), likens this attitude to the Eastern Indian Ayurvedic approach, as opposed to traditional Western medicine: "When clients come in to see me and they ask me, 'What should I eat?' the first thing I want to know is, who is the 'I'? Who is the person sitting before me? Traditional Western medicine asks, 'What is the disease?' Ayurvedic medicine asks, 'Who is the person who has the disease?'"

In the long run, what you eat is up to you. Everyone has a dirty little eating secret. For many people, it involves sweets and ice cream, but one client of mine used to sneak downstairs at four o'clock in the morning to snack on sardines and biscuits. You may be able to hide these secrets from your friends and family, but you can't hide them from your body.

If you want to help your body reach peak performance, you'll have to consider yourself a scientific experiment for the rest of your life. You try one thing and then another. You combine these foods with these supplements. You add a little exercise. You eliminate one food and substitute another. You keep experimenting until you find the combination that works right just for you.

Your purpose is to find the balance of elements that keeps you healthy. And since your body is constantly changing, your nutritional requirements will change as well. When you find the right combination for you, stay with it as long as it makes you feel fit and healthy. If, after a year, or five or ten, your hormones begin to change somewhat, or your lifestyle or stress levels change, continue your experimentation. Adjust your exercise regimen, make some new food choices, take a different supplement. As you read on and assimilate the guidelines that are being laid down here, follow this simple scientific principle: Test it out, see if it works, then make your decisions on the basis of your findings.

LAYING DOWN THE GROUND RULES

That said, there are some general ground rules that you can follow to achieve a body in balance.

Reduce or Eliminate Unnecessary Stimulants

To follow this rule, you'll have to make some sacrifices. You know what they are: caffeine, tobacco, excessive alcohol, sugar, refined carbohydrates—all the things discussed in chapters 1 through 6. I'm not telling you never to have these things again. I have an occasional cup of coffee, chocolate pudding, or side order of chips. What I am recommending is that you regard these items as condiments, elements that can be added as embellishments to your menu but are not your sole source of calories.

Eat Breakfast

For years, your grandmother has been telling you that breakfast is the most important meal of the day. She may be right. Since most people stay up for several hours after they eat dinner, then sleep for six to eight hours, a big chunk of time goes by without supplying food to the body. When you wake up, your blood sugar is low and you're in need of refueling. Think about the times you have rushed to work, or to an important meeting, without any breakfast. You probably felt anxious and irritable, as well as unprepared. Your brain didn't seem to be making the connections it should. Facts that were easily retrievable the night before disappeared, and the only thing you could think about was food. Studies have shown that people who eat a nutritional breakfast (that means including several food groups, not just carbohydrates and caffeine) tend to be more productive during the day, as well as less hungry and less likely to overeat later on.

Eat Five or Six Times a Day

Imagine this scenario: You're driving along in your car when you notice that the needle is fast approaching empty. You're in unfamiliar territory and don't know where the next petrol station is. You know you can't reach your destination without adding more fuel. As you watch the needle drop, your tension and anxiety levels increase. If you're lucky, you get to a petrol station in time, but not before you've made yourself sick with worry. Or else you find yourself stranded on the motorway, fresh out of fuel and luck.

Your body, like your car, cannot go long distances without fuel. As your fuel level begins to drop, your tension and anxiety levels increase, and your ability to function well decreases. Unfortunately, we have been conditioned to eat only three meals a day, no matter how many hours are in between each meal. If you're dieting, you've probably been told that eating between meals is what made you fat in the first place. But it's not eating between meals that makes you fat; it's eating biscuits, chocolate bars, and crisps between meals that makes you fat.

If you eat a protein-based snack between meals (as outlined in the following chapters), you keep your fuel supply on an even keel throughout the day. Snacking works for your body in two ways. First, there is a hormone in the brain called *galanin* that regulates the body's desire for fat. When the body begins to break down body fat, galanin is released. The longer you go between meals, the more body fat is broken down and the more galanin is produced. The longer the amount of time that goes by between meals, the more the body craves fat. If you cut down that amount of time, the body produces less galanin, and the desire for fat is cut short.

Second, snacking reduces the hunger factor. It's just common sense: The hungrier you are, the more you will eat, whether you need all that food or not. If you've eaten lunch at noon, and dinner isn't until seven or eight, your body will be running out of fuel, your appetite will be out of control, and you're more than likely to overeat. If you've had a protein-rich snack at three or four, however, you simply won't be as hungry.

Drink Water

Water is the source of life and the most important nutrient in your body. You can't get enough of the stuff. Drink up to eight to ten glasses a day. It is interesting to note that a decrease in optimum hydration of as little as 3 percent can lead to a measurable reduction in strength and speed.

Reduce or Eliminate Flour, Wheat, and Gluten

Foods with a high gluten content can lead to food allergies in people sensitive to flour, and they may contribute to weight gain owing to water retention and cravings. Gluten overload (especially when accompanied by high-fat and low-protein diets) can cause such illnesses as yeast infections, PMS, and chronic fatigue syndrome. Because of this, I usually recommend diets low in wheat.

Consider All Meals Interchangeable

Open your mind to new ways of eating. In the United States, people have strong ideas about what foods constitute breakfast, lunch, and dinner. Breakfast consists of cereal, a muffin, a bagel, an occasional egg, or (for a special treat) pancakes or waffles. Lunch is a light meal, perhaps a sandwich or a salad. Dinner is the largest meal and usually the most variable, ranging from the standard meat and potatoes meal to exotic French cuisine.

In the Balance program, there are no hard and fast rules about what you should have for breakfast, or what constitutes a good lunch or dinner. A breakfast option is as good as a snack is as good as a dinner meal. If you want to have a breakfast suggestion for dinner or a lunch meal for breakfast, that's perfectly okay. As long as you are eating meals that are appropriate for your metabolic type and have them when you need them, you can call them whatever you like.

Be Prepared

Remember the story of Susannah, the student who ran into trouble when confronted with the stress of university life? The reason she ran into trouble was that she let herself get overwhelmed by a pressure-packed situation and an unfamiliar schedule. Her usual meal breaks didn't coincide with her class schedule, so that by the time she got to eat, she was too hungry to make healthy choices.

She didn't have to change her entire schedule to keep herself on track. All she had to do to turn her situation around was to prepare for her day in advance. Knowing that she wouldn't have a chance to grab an appropriate snack between breakfast and lunch, she began to prepare foods the night before and bring them to class. She found she could bring her lunch in her rucksack, or have a salad in the canteen and make healthy choices. She also scheduled a shopping trip once a week so that she wouldn't be caught pulling an all-nighter with nothing to do except order out for pizza.

You can prepare yourself mentally as well. Some days are not easy to plan. You don't know exactly where you'll be or how long you'll be there. You're rushing between appointments, it's time for a snack, and the only food source you see is the sandwich shop. You'll have to eat on the run. The easiest solution seems to be to run into the shop and grab a bag of crisps. We all know this type of situation is ripe for making bad food choices. So why not carry a mental list of "emergency" food options? Instead of a bag of crisps look for a small container of yogurt or cottage cheese with fruit. Pick up an apple or a pear. Make your list at home, when you're not in a rush to do anything and when you're not hungry or stressed out. When you find yourself in a hurry with choices to make, you will have a selection of healthy choices to choose from.

Choose the Best Quality Foods Possible

It would be wonderful if everyone could afford the best quality organic meats, fruits, and vegetables. However, organic foods are not always available, and when they are, they are often outrageously expensive. If these foods are within your budget, go for it. If they're not, don't worry about it. Choose what you can afford. Look for lean meats and poultry. Be sure to check expiration dates on everything you buy from the supermarket. Buy fresh fruits and vegetables—the fresher the better—whenever you can. Make an attempt to eat foods that are grown, plucked, or harvested rather than those that are boxed, frozen, or canned. Bodybuilders call this "eating clean." Try to buy what is in season. It's also better to eat whole foods rather than those that have been precut or sliced. You lose vitamins by buying things that are sliced, diced, or shredded. If you can't find the fresh vegetable you want, frozen is your next best option. Avoid canned fruits and vegetables, if possible; they retain the least amount of nutrients. Here's a sure way to eat cleaner: Cut back on the number of foods you eat that come packaged with a list of ingredients on the wrapper.

LET'S TALK ABOUT FAT

If you notice, I did not list "Give up fat" as one of the ground rules. In fact, I might just as well add a ground rule that states: *Fat is not your enemy*. The notion that fat is to blame for all our nutritional ills was given great credence by Nathan Pritikin in the early 1970s. Pritikin was not a doctor, but when he was diagnosed with a heart condition in 1955, he spent the next twenty-five years studying other cultures of the world to find those with low rates of heart disease. He found cultures in Africa, New Guinea, Ecuador, and Mexico in which the population exists on diets of about 10 percent fat. These peoples also had a high percentage of complex carbohydrates in their diets and not much protein.

Pritikin developed the theory, therefore, that Americans should also live on a low-fat, low-protein, high-carbohydrate diet. Although this may have been a good solution for a select group of people, it was not good for everyone. As for Pritikin's examples of cultures with low-fat diets and little heart disease, there are many groups of people around the world who eat higher percentages of fat (including Eskimos, with a diet that is 70 percent fat, and Greeks and Italians, whose diets are about 40 percent fat) and have low rates of heart disease.

It seems like such a logical concept: Eat less fat and you become less fat. Unfortunately, that theory doesn't hold up. The public and—much more damaging—the food producers have latched onto the "low-fat, no-fat" approach to food consumption as the ultimate answer to weight loss and a healthy heart. The past few years, however, have brought about a new understanding of the role of fats in our diet.

It takes energy to digest, absorb, and assimilate the various nutrients from any food we take in. This process burns more calories from protein and carbohydrate than it does with fat. About 23 out of every 100 calories from protein, for example, are burned in the process of absorbing nutrients. Fat, on the other hand, comes into the body almost in the form in which it can be stored. We only use about 3 calories out of every 100 calories of fat to adapt it to the form in which it resides on your hips. If in one day you ate 2,000 calories of fat, it would probably make you heavier than if you ate 2,000 calories of carbohydrate or protein.

The problem with the Pritikin diet and other diets that followed from his philosophy is that Pritikin based his theory on two false premises: that all people are alike (therefore, what is good for one culture is good for another) and that all fats are alike. However, research now tells us that neither of these premises is true.

All foods are eventually broken down into their smallest components for use by the body. Carbohydrates break down into sugars, and proteins break down into amino acids. When fat is used by our bodies, it is broken down into fatty acids. There are two kinds of fats in our diets: saturated and unsaturated. Because saturated fat has a large amount of hydrogen attached to it, it is usually solid at room temperature; it is found in animal fats and in some tropical oils such as coconut and palm.

Figure 7.1A

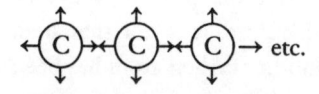

Imagine a line of carbon atoms with four "arms" branching out from it (see Figure 7.1A). One arm is always holding onto another carbon atom, leaving two or three arms free. If each free arm is attached to a hydrogen atom, the fatty acid is saturated (see Figure 7.1B).

Figure 7.1B

Figure 7.1C

Figure 7.1D

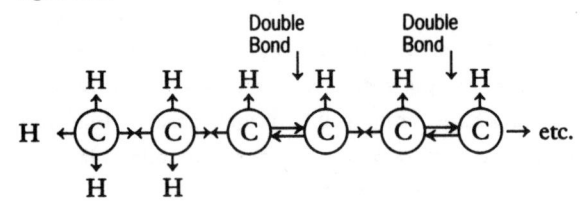

If, however, one of the arms is brought across to connect to another carbon atom in a chain, there is one place for a hydrogen atom to become attached. Therefore, it is not saturated. What is called a double bond to another carbon atom has been created. If one of these bonds is in a chain, the fat is *mono*unsaturated (see Figure 7.1C). If there are more than one of these bonds in a chain, the fat is *poly*unsaturated (see Figure 7.1D).

The Good, the Bad, and the Trans Fatty

All of these fats are necessary, to varying degrees, for our health. Saturated fats, which have gotten such a bad reputation over the years, provide our bodies with a good source of energy when we are low on fuel, serve as "shock absorbers" for our internal organs, and insulate us against the cold. Fats also help to keep cell membranes fluid so that, for example, red blood cells can squeeze through capillaries. Like every other food I've discussed, saturated fats are harmful only when they are consumed in excess. It's not the saturated fat in a small amount of butter that's going to do us in; it's the great gobs of it that we spread on bread, muffins, and potatoes. It's not the steak with a small amount of fat in it that's harmful; it's the deep-fried foods. It's all the cakes, biscuits, cereals, and baked goods that are made with highly saturated palm and coconut oil or partially hydrogenated vegetable oil.

Hydrogenated oils are oils to which hydrogen has been artificially added at extremely high temperatures to solidify them and give them longer shelf lives. Margarine is probably the most well-known partially hydrogenated product. Although it was created to be a healthier alternative to the saturated fat found in butter, margarine unfortunately turned out to be an *un*healthy alternative. The process of hydrogenating the fat causes it to change its molecular structure into what is called a *trans fatty acid*, and trans fatty acid has a harmful effect on cholesterol levels. Ann Louise Gittleman, in her book *Your Body Knows Best*, explains that "the consumption of trans fatty acids *lowers* the level of the protective, or good, HDL cholesterol while *raising* that of the oxidizing, or bad LDL cholesterol. Consuming foods that contain trans fats actually raises total cholesterol levels more than eating foods with saturated fats." She goes so far as to say that "unnatural trans fats are *biochemically incompatible* with the human body, and have no business being used as food." Both the dairy and meat-producing industries are happy that there is no longer a nutritional diatribe against their products. That doesn't mean you should eat steak at every meal and put butter on everything. It means it's perfectly all right to have red meat once or perhaps twice a week and to spread a small amount of butter on your vegetables as a seasoning.

Essential Fatty Acids

Saturated fats do not tell the whole fat story. There are other fats that are helpful to the body. In fact, there are two fatty acids that are so important we cannot function properly without them. These are called essential fatty acids (EFAs). The body cannot manufacture these essential fatty acids; we have to get them through our diets (and sometimes through supplements).

The two essential fatty acids are linolenic (also called alpha-linolenic) and linoleic. Linolenic acid is an omega-3 acid. Chemists use the term *omega-3* for a fat that has its first double bond in the third position (see Figure 7.1E). Linoleic acid is an omega-6 acid, which means it has its first double bond in the sixth position (see Figure 7.1F).

Now, if that isn't confusing enough, there are further subdivisions. Omega-3 produces both eicosapentaenoic acid (EPA) and docosahexaenoic acid (DHA). Omega-6 produces gamma-linoleic acid (GLA). I discuss each of these in chapter 11. Suffice it to say that all of these acids are necessary for body functions, including the production of sex and adrenal hormones, and for the control of cell growth. They also help dissolve body fats into body fluids, aid in maintaining body temperature, and distribute vitamins A, D, E, and K throughout the body.

Recent research has shown omega-3 oils to be particularly helpful in reducing the risk of heart diseases. Omega-3 oils are found largely in cold-water or deep-ocean fish, such as halibut, cod, salmon, tuna, sardines, and mackerel. In 1997, physicians at Brigham and Women's Hospital in Boston published a study they had completed in which twenty thousand male doctors were followed over a period of years. Doctors who ate at least

The Balance

Figure 7.1E

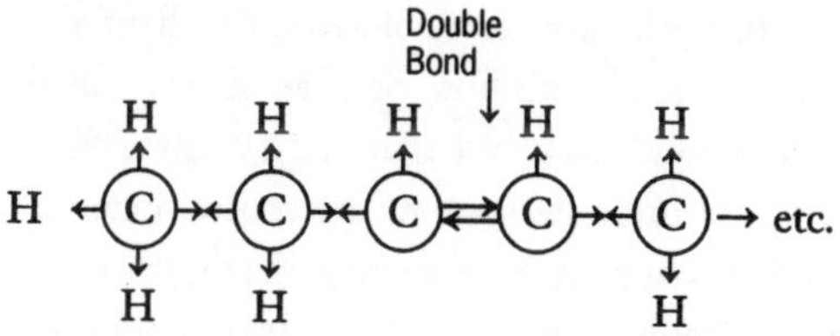

Figure 7.1F

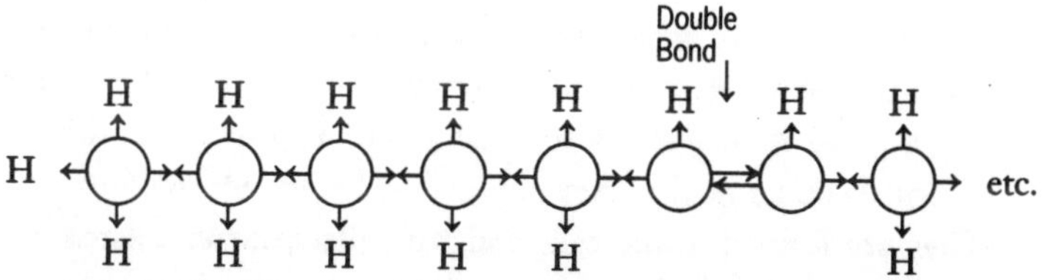

Carbon and hydrogen atoms link together to form saturated and unsaturated fats. The various ways these atoms are linked define the types of fats we consume.

one fish meal a week reduced their risk of sudden death from heart attack by 60 percent!

One of the reasons for this is that EFAs are cholesterol carriers; that is, they help move bad cholesterol (LDL) out of the body. If there is not enough EFA in the body, the cholesterol becomes attached to fat molecules, which usually end up coating arterial walls (thereby increasing the risk of heart disease).

Omega-6 oils, which are found in green leafy vegetables and in flaxseed, safflower, borage, and evening primrose oils, stimulate fat-burning tissue in the body, encouraging calories to be burned for energy instead of being stored as fat.

The Eicosanoid Connection

There is another even more basic reason for maintaining the proper amount of fat in the body. In fact, there are millions of tiny, fleeting reasons, and they are called *eicosanoids*. Eicosanoids are manufactured by the cells and control virtually all of the body's functions. Barry Sears, author of *The Zone*, called eicosanoids "superhormones" and said that they control "the cardiovascular system, the immune system, the central nervous system, the reproductive system, and so on. When you get right down to it, eicosanoids are in charge of nothing less than keeping us alive and well. Without eicosanoids, life as we know it would be impossible."

Eicosanoids are a recent discovery in the scientific community (they've been researched seriously only since the early 1970s), and there's still a lot that is not known about them. Scientists do know that they are extremely difficult to pinpoint. They are formed in the cells and have life spans calculated in miniseconds. As part of the balanced body system, there are two types of eicosanoids: good ones and bad ones. Both serve purposes in our bodies. "Good" eicosanoids help keep veins and arteries clear and unconstricted. "Bad" eicosanoids help clot blood when we cut ourselves. They are labeled *bad* because disease occurs when there is an imbalance, with more bad eicosanoids than good ones.

According to Sears, "virtually every disease state—whether it be heart disease, cancer, or autoimmune disease like arthritis and multiple sclerosis—can be viewed at the molecular level as the body simply making more bad eicosanoids and fewer good ones." The goal is not to eliminate bad eicosanoids, but to be sure that there are always more good guys than bad guys.

This is where essential fatty acids and what we eat come back into the picture. Eicosanoids are made from essential fatty acids, and the only way we get essential fatty acids into our bodies is through what we eat. Getting enough fatty acids is only the first step. Once those fatty acids are ingested, we want the majority of them to be turned into good eicosanoids. The process is a bit like getting supplies into war-torn Bosnia. There are not too many hurdles getting supplies to the nearest airport. It's when you want to distribute the supplies to the people who really need them that you run into problems.

You may have enough essential fatty acids in your diet, but there may be many things in your diet that mitigate against the proper distribution of these acids, thereby blocking the formation of good eicosanoids. The biggest barrier is the presence of large amounts of insulin. If you are eating a high-carbohydrate, high-sugar diet, you are producing large amounts of insulin and suppressing the production of eicosanoids.

The Cholesterol Connection

There is another side to the "fat is the enemy" controversy. We have been taught over the past few decades that foods such as red meat, fats, and especially eggs contain cholesterol and therefore should be avoided. But the latest data show that, once again, we have been throwing the baby out with the bathwater.

Cholesterol, like fat, is essential to our survival. It helps produce vitamin D and helps the body repair damaged cell membranes. It is used as a building block of estrogen and testosterone, and it is necessary for the production of cortisone. Approximately 80 percent of the cholesterol in our bodies is produced by the cells themselves. Cholesterol, like eicosanoids, is divided into the "good" and the "bad." Good cholesterol is high-density lipoprotein (HDL), which is carried to the liver, where it is broken down into bile and eventually eliminated from the body. Bad cholesterol is low-density lipoprotein (LDL), which carries fat and cholesterol throughout the body and deposits them in various spots, including the arteries.

If you don't have enough cholesterol in your body, your cells will produce more or will grab some floating by in the bloodstream. If you greatly reduce the amount of cholesterol you're ingesting, the body will only produce more. So the warnings we have been given about eating cholesterol don't seem to hold true; eating foods that contain cholesterol doesn't, in fact, add much cholesterol to our bloodstream.

A report in the June 1997 issue of the *American Journal of Clinical Nutrition* "lays to rest a long-standing public health controversy regarding the relevance of dietary cholesterol on blood cholesterol levels." The study, by Drs. Wanda Howell and Donald McNamara at the University of Arizona, analyzed 224 scientific trials on cholesterol that were conducted over the past twenty-five years. Their conclusion? According to Dr. McNamara, "the restriction of foods rich in dietary cholesterol is now proven to have little—if any—scientific justification." Adds Dr. Howell, "For most people, the cholesterol they eat does not raise their blood cholesterol. So, healthy individuals with normal cholesterol levels should now feel free to enjoy foods like eggs in their diet every day."

Saturated fat, however, has been shown to raise blood cholesterol levels. Margarine contains no cholesterol, which is why it was created in the first place, but it does contain the artificially saturated trans fatty acids. Therefore, margarine is probably more of a hazard to your heart than butter, even though butter contains cholesterol.

Once again, insulin enters into the equation. When you eat a high-carbohydrate, high-sugar diet, you increase the level of insulin in the body. Insulin signals the cells to produce more cholesterol. When the body produces more cholesterol, there is no need for cells to grab the excess floating by in the bloodstream. That excess is then free to build up where you don't want it, specifically in the arteries. If you follow the food plan for your metabolic type, you will automatically reduce the level of insulin, and therefore the level of excess cholesterol, in your body.

CALORIES, PORTION SIZE, AND PERCENTAGES

In the next three chapters, you will learn what to eat for your specific metabolic type. Although you will find guidelines for foods that will work best for you, you won't find, in most cases, caloric restrictions or complicated numerical comparisons of carbohydrates to proteins to fats. However, I have included portion sizes in some instances.

The Balance is about developing a lifelong plan for healthy living. It seems unrealistic to expect that you will count every calorie in every meal every day of your life. Nor do I expect you to carry a calculator around with you to figure out the ratio of a potato to a piece of chicken. When you begin to eat according to your metabolic guidelines, you'll be able to determine for yourself the right volumes naturally. And as you add exercise and supplements into your routine, you will make even more adjustments.

We don't eat too much because we're not counting calories. We eat too much because we're in a stressful situation, because we only have fifteen minutes to wolf down a meal, because it's been too long between meals. We end up eating higher calorie foods, fast foods, and foods that contain high percentages of sugars and carbohydrates. Then we end up hungrier. When you begin to organize yourself around the appropriate guidelines, your appetite will balance itself out and you will naturally gravitate to the amount of calories you need in a day.

This, too, will take time. If you've been eating in a haphazard manner all your life, you'll be resistant to making these changes. You may be enthusiastic for a few weeks and then find yourself slipping into old habits. Enthusiasm is an elusive animal. It happened to me when I was training for the New York City Marathon. I began training in January, thrilled to be out running in the park and totally focused on my goal. But the race was ten months away. I hit points in my training when my speed seemed to be decreasing or I couldn't get past a certain distance. I was repeating my training routine exactly and not making progress. It seemed October was never going to get here, and why was I doing this anyway?

That's when I knew I had to make some changes, go back and reevaluate my training from the level I was now at. What works for a beginner doesn't necessarily work when your body begins to adapt to conditioning. You can't count on enthusiasm to keep you going. You need to ask yourself constantly, How do I feel? Am I comfortable with the foods I'm eating? Am I following the guidelines to good eating?

8

DOWN TO A SLOW CRAWL: REVVING UP A SLOW BURNER

DOING THE SLOW BURN

You took the test and you've come out a slow burner. You're in good company. About 70 percent of Westerners are slow burners. Just what is a slow burner anyway? You've had glimpses throughout the previous chapters, but it's time for a more detailed description.

First, we need to remember that the body is made up of many different systems of checks and balances. Human beings (and most other living creatures as well) are designed so that parts of our bodies are in constant opposition to other parts. Some parts are made to take in the nutrients we need to survive; others are made to eliminate waste. Some parts are made to help us react spontaneously to immediate danger; others are designed to help us make reasonable decisions over a long time span. Our bodies function best when we achieve a state of balance—when all our systems are working at equal strength and capacity.

Unfortunately for us, in today's fast-food, overprocessed, toxin-laden environment, that hardly ever happens.

The nervous system, which is the part of our body that oversees our metabolic functioning, is one of the systems of checks and balances. It is divided into two categories: the voluntary and the involuntary nervous systems. The voluntary nervous system allows us to do things on a conscious level, like make decisions, walk, and talk. These are things over which we have control. We can choose to do these things or not to do them.

The involuntary system has control over functions that go on without any choice on our part. It takes care of things that go on in our body automatically, such as heart rate, respiration, blood pressure, digestion, and glandular function. We can modify certain aspects of this system (like purposely slowing down our rate of respiration or speeding up our metabolism), but we don't have a choice about whether or not these functions will occur.

The involuntary nervous system, which is the master regulator of metabolism, is broken down further to include the sympathetic and parasympathetic systems. For those fortunate few mixed burners, these two systems balance each other out. The sympathetic nervous system (which gives us speed and anger and heightened awareness in dangerous situations) is balanced by the parasympathetic system (which gives us calmness, thoughtfulness, and the ability to return to normal when danger has passed). For most people, however, these two systems usually are not in balance, and one is dominant over the other.

Although we do not have direct control over these systems—we can't will our thyroid to change its metabolic functioning, nor can we will the pancreas to produce less insulin—we can influence how efficiently these hormone producers work. We can exert our influence by making changes in our diet, exercise, and supplementation.

The sympathetic nervous system controls, among other things, the adrenal glands and the thyroid. I talk more about these in the next chapter because they are the glands that most influence fast burners.

If you are a slow burner, your metabolic rate is dominated by the parasympathetic nervous system, which is controlled by, among other things, the parathyroid gland and the pancreas (see Figure 8.1). The parathyroid gland is responsible for regulating calcium and phosphate levels in the body. The pancreas is responsible for the secretion of various hormones, such as insulin and glucagon, and the digestive enzymes. When the parathyroid gland and the pancreas are overactive, they slow down your ability to use nutrients efficiently, thereby preventing you from obtaining optimum health and energy levels.

A SLOW BURNER IS . . .

Following is a list of generalizations that can be made about slow burners. You must remember, however, that although you may be dominated by one set of glands or another, the opposing glandular systems are still functioning to varying degrees. Our bodies contain the glands and organs that produce all three types of burners; therefore, although an overall description of the slow burner may suit you, there are probably some characteristics that fit you to a tee, while others may not apply to you at all.

Figure 8.1

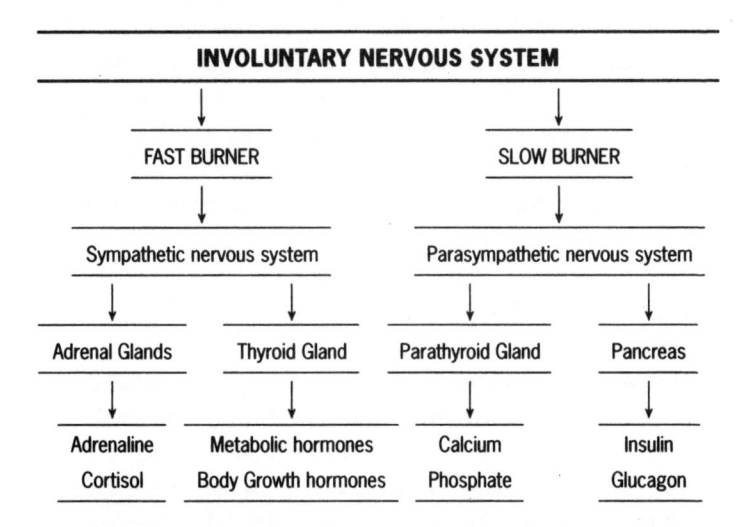

INVOLUNTARY NERVOUS SYSTEM			
FAST BURNER		SLOW BURNER	
Sympathetic nervous system		Parasympathetic nervous system	
Adrenal Glands	Thyroid Gland	Parathyroid Gland	Pancreas
Adrenaline Cortisol	Metabolic hormones Body Growth hormones	Calcium Phosphate	Insulin Glucagon

The involuntary nervous system is composed of the sympathetic and parasympathetic nervous systems. Slow burners are dominated by the parasympathetic nervous system, and fast burners are dominated by the sympathetic nervous system

- If you are moving towards the extreme of slow oxidation, you probably feel tired fairly often. You may tire easily after a minimum of exertion. You may experience hypoglycemia, or low blood sugar, caused by too much insulin, which can also cause fatigue.
- Another condition related to high insulin levels is called *hyperinsulinemia*, which is the excess production of insulin created by an overactive pancreas (and by too many carbohydrates in the diet). The pancreas produces both insulin and glucagon (another part of the system of checks and balances). One function of insulin is to send fat into storage, so that the body has a supply to use when it can't get enough to eat. The function of glucagon is to help release that stored body fat, allowing the body to use it for energy. If the pancreas is

producing more insulin, it is producing less glucagon. The stored body fat then remains in storage, and the law of supply and demand takes over: Since you can't call on the supplies you already have in storage, the body demands that you bring in more from outside sources, and you crave more carbohydrates; eating more carbohydrates creates more insulin, which lowers the amount of glucagon produced, which decreases the use of stored fat . . . and on and on.

- This cycle of too much insulin and not enough glucagon naturally leads to weight gain. If you are a slow burner and you are overweight, most of your weight is gained in the hips, buttocks, and thighs, creating a pear-shaped silhouette. (Overweight fast burners tend to gain weight in the abdominal region, and are more of an apple shape.) David Watts, author of *Trace Elements and Other Essential Nutrients*, offers this formula to determine if you have an apple- or pear-shaped body: Measure your hips and waist. Then divide your waist measurement by your hip measurement. If the result is 0.75 or less you have a pear-shaped body type. If the result is greater than 0.75 you have a tendency toward an apple shape.
- Because slow metabolism decreases circulation rates, you may also be sensitive to cold, especially in your hands and feet.
- Slow burners are often insomniacs, waking several times during the night. Even if you sleep for ten or twelve hours, however, you may wake up feeling tired. This, too, is the result of low energy. You need energy to reach the rapid eye movement (REM) stage of sleep. If you don't reach that stage, you will not be fully rested, and you will feel chronically fatigued.

Here are some general psychological and physiological traits of slow burners:

- Calmness
- Cautiousness
- Coolness
- Dislike of exercise
- Emotional stability
- Ease in falling asleep; may have trouble remaining asleep
- Fast clotting time
- Difficulty getting going in the morning
- Good digestion
- Good endurance levels
- High calcium levels
- High stress tolerance
- Low blood pressure
- Low sodium levels
- Makes decisions slowly
- May have bouts of depression
- Moist eyes
- Poor concentration
- Seldom gets angry
- Slow heartbeat
- Strong appetite
- Has vivid dreams, easily recalled

Here are some physical conditions and diseases slow burners are prone to:

- Allergies
- Anorexia
- Asthma
- Chronic fatigue syndrome
- Colds, coughs
- Diabetes (adult onset)
- Eczema

- Gastric ulcers
- Hay fever
- Hypoglycemia
- Hypothyroidism
- Lupus
- Osteoarthritis (arthritis that is limited to one area rather than systemic)
- PMS
- Vital infections
- Yeast infections

ON THE MENU

When I work with a client who is a slow burner, I lay out a food plan to be used as a guideline, including foods that are most important for each type.

The foods on this chart will help you speed up your sluggish metabolism, give you more energy, and build up your resistance to the diseases to which you may otherwise be prone. Of course, I haven't included every possible food item on this list, but I've tried to be as inclusive as possible (see Figure 8.2).

This food plan contains eight major categories:

1. Animal protein: seafood, hoofed animals, and poultry
2. Vegetable protein: soy products like tofu and tempeh
3. Vegetables: fibrous and starchy
4. Fruits
5. Grains and grain products
6. Fats and oils
7. Beverages
8. Designer foods

Figure 8.2

FOODS FOR SLOW BURNERS

ANIMAL PROTEIN			VEGETABLE PROTEIN	VEGETABLES		FRUITS	GRAINS & GRAIN PRODUCTS	FATS & OILS	BEVERAGES	DESIGNER FOODS
Hoofed	Poultry	Seafood		Fibrous	Starchy					
Beef (lean)	Chicken Eggs Turkey Dairy Low-fat cheese Low-fat milk Low-fat yogurt	Catfish Cod Flounder Haddock Perch Scrod Sole Swordfish Tuna Turbot	Tofu Tempeh	Bean sprouts Beetroot Broccoli Brussels sprouts Cabbage Carrots Celery Cucumbers Green beans Kale Lettuce Okra Onions Peppers Spinach	Potato Squash Sweet potatoes	Apple Apricot Banana Berries Cantaloupe melon Cherry Grapefruit Honeydew melon Orange Peach Pear Plum	Brown rice Kasha Oatmeal Quinoa	Olive oil Sesame oil Canola oil Flaxseed oil Butter	Herbal tea Vegetable juice Water	Designer shakes Protein bars

Animal Protein: Seafood, Hoofed Animals, and Poultry

All metabolic types (which means all human beings) need protein in their diet. The general rule for slow burners is to stay with the lighter proteins: chicken, turkey, and fish such as flounder, sole, cod, haddock, turbot, and perch. Because of the health benefits of cold-water and deep-ocean fish, however, you should try to have a minimum of one meal a week that includes such fish as tuna, salmon, halibut, and sardines. If you have tuna from a can, make it water-packed. You can have red meat, but keep it lean, and try to keep it to one or two servings a week. These proteins can be broiled, boiled, roasted, baked, or grilled. Avoid frying if possible.

Limit dairy products to two servings a day. Because dairy is a calcium-rich food source, and slow burners are known to have high calcium levels, adding more will only slow down your metabolism further. Look for low-fat cheeses, milk, and yogurt.

Vegetarian Protein: Soy Products like Tofu and Tempeh

Tofu, tempeh, and other soy products, found in products such as soyburgers and soy frankfurters, can be good substitutes for animal protein. The problem is that you have to eat large portions of tofu to equal the amount of animal protein you need. If you are a vegetarian, you should try to add one or more fish meals and/or some eggs and cheese to your diet.

Vegetables: Fibrous and Starchy

Ever since you were old enough to eat whole foods, your mother has been trying to get you to eat your vegetables—and with good reason. Besides providing many essential vitamins and minerals, vegetables also provide fiber. Fiber aids in the digestion of foods and the elimination of waste. It also helps to stabilize blood sugar by slowing down the rate at which you absorb the carbohydrates you eat.

You should include at least four servings of fibrous vegetables a day (4 ounces/115 grams cooked or 8 ounces/225 grams raw is considered one serving). However, you may have as many servings of these vegetables as you like. Try having some for breakfast to give you a good start for the day.

Consumption of starchy vegetables should be limited to one or two servings a day. Try having 4 ounces/115 grams of squash, two small red potatoes, or half a sweet potato.

Fruits

Fruits, like vegetables, are good sources of vitamins. Unlike vegetables, however, they are high in fructose, a simple sugar that converts easily into glucose. The glucose stimulates the production of insulin and blocks the production of glucagon. Too much fruit, therefore, can keep your body from using stored fat. You should also be careful about buying foods that are sweetened with fructose. Many people assume that foods, especially snack foods, sweetened with fruit juice or fructose are healthier than those sweetened with sugar. In reality, these sweeteners can wreak havoc with your blood sugar levels.

Slow burners should have two to three servings of fruit a day. The fruits usually recommended for slow burners are apples, pears, all types of berries, oranges, and grapefruits. Citrus fruits are more likely to stimulate metabolism, so they are not recommended to fast burners. Another fruit that is recommended more often for slow than for fast burners is the banana. Both bananas and citrus fruits are high in potassium, a mineral that is found in lower levels in slow burners.

Grains and Grain Products

Starchy carbohydrates should be limited. If you are trying to lose weight, they should be avoided altogether for a while. That includes breads, rolls or baps, muffins, pastas, cold cereals, cakes, and biscuits. I recommend that slow burners in general stay away from the more "provocative" carbohydrates and choose instead 4 ounces/115 grams of basmati rice or cooked kasha, quinoa, or oatmeal. If you are going to have bread, try a multigrain loaf.

Fats and Oils

Since slow burners have increased levels of insulin and decreased levels of glucagon, and the utilization of stored body fat is impaired, they should not add too much more fat into the system. If you're a slow burner, it's a good idea to limit your intake of fats to about two tablespoons per day. This includes flaxseed or sesame oil for salads and olive or canola oil for cooking. Use butter sparingly on potatoes and other vegetables.

Beverages

Here's my advice about drinking water: *Drink as much as you can.* Most people don't drink enough during the day. We need at least eight glasses a day to help eliminate fat that is not used for fuel. That includes tap water, filtered water, and plain or flavored mineral waters. A glass or two a day of vegetable juice can be a tasty addition to your liquid intake, but beware of too much sodium. You can get low- or no-sodium versions of vegetable juice and add your own salt if you feel you need it.

Fruit juice is another story. When you eat a piece of fruit, it converts quickly into glucose and then into fat. When you *drink* a piece of fruit in the form of juice, that process becomes even faster (and you're not getting the benefit of the fiber in the fruit), so that you suffer from the "peak-and-valley" syndrome of a quick sugar high, followed by a fast drop to the bottom.

Avoid using coffee as a source of water, for all the reasons discussed earlier. Tea has less of a caffeine effect than coffee; however, you should not drink regular (black) tea in excess of one or two cups a day. Herbal teas are, for the most part, benign. Feel free to choose a cup of herbal tea as part of your daily liquid intake.

Limit your intake of fizzy drinks. Both diet and regular sodas contain phosphoric acid, which interferes with the absorption of calcium. Although slow burners usually have high levels of calcium, the mineral does no good if it is not absorbed where it is needed.

Designer Foods: Shakes and Power Bars

These shake mixes and power bars are readily available in most health food stores. For both fast and slow oxidizers, shakes may be a powerful breakfast option. You'll find out how to use them as you read on. I recommend whey peptide beverages (whey is a byproduct of milk). A favorite at my center is Designer Protein by Next Nutrition. These shakes are low in fat and carbohydrates, and high in protein. The Next Nutrition company also makes a powder called ISO, which is a combination of whey peptides and other ingredients with higher carbohydrate and fat contents.

You can experiment and see which you like best. You can mix the powder with water to make a shake, or add it to foods like yogurt or cereals to enhance their protein value. One interesting thing about whey peptide powders is that they have been found to have an inhibiting effect on appetite and cravings by causing cholecystokinin (CCK) levels (the chemicals that tell you you're full) to be released sooner rather than later.

If you're in a hurry and in need of a quick energy snack, I recommend "power bars," which you can find in many supermarkets and health food shops. Read the label; not all power bars are alike. You want the one with the lowest amount of fat and sugar, and the highest protein level.

The Balance

STRUCTURING YOUR DAY

As you know from reading the guidelines to good eating set out in the previous chapter, your day should consist of five meals, three larger and two smaller ones. This is less important for slow burners than for fast or mixed burners, because slow burners use up fuel at a slower pace. You may not get as hungry during the day as fast burners do, but don't let yourself go too long without eating or you're likely to eat too much at the next meal. Remember that the following meal suggestions are interchangeable; if you feel like having breakfast for dinner or vice versa, go right ahead.

Breakfast Suggestions

Every day should start off with a healthy breakfast. Breakfast should always contain protein to give your day the proper energy foundation. If you enjoy fruit in the morning, have one-half grapefruit or 4 ounces/115 grams of a variety of berries. Use fresh fruit, not canned or frozen, whenever possible. Here are some breakfast options a slow burner might consider:

- *The quick shake.* If you're in a hurry or are not normally a breakfast eater, this shake takes just minutes to prepare and can be a great energy booster. In the blender, mix one scoop of Ultra Clear and two scoops of Designer Protein with six ounces of water. Add in one tablespoon of flaxseed oil. You can also add 4 ounces/115 grams of peaches, pears, strawberries, blueberries, or raspberries.
- *The three-egg vegetable omelet.* Cook three eggs in one-half to one tablespoon of olive oil (if you're concerned about the fat content, use one whole egg and the whites of two eggs). Add in 2 ounces/50 grams each of some of your favorite vegetables, like mushrooms, broccoli, peppers, and onions.

- *The cheese omelet.* The recipe is the same as for the three-egg vegetable omelet, with the addition of 2 ounces/50 grams of low-fat cheese.
- *Poached eggs and spinach.* Poach two eggs (easier than ever if you use a microwave poacher) and pour them out over a bed of steamed spinach.
- *Eggs and sausage.* Two scrambled eggs (cooked in olive oil) and two turkey sausages.
- *Eggs and mince "hash."* Sauté 4 ounces/115 grams of lean mince in a skillet, using one tablespoon of olive oil. Add in two whole eggs, some of your favorite vegetables, and scramble together. Serve over two slices of tomato.
- *Oatmeal and eggs.* As a general rule, it is better not to have starchy carbohydrate for breakfast. But if you need an occasional change of menu, have 12 ounces/340 grams of oatmeal and one poached or hard-boiled egg.
- *Fish and veggies.* Four ounces/115 grams of cooked fish or half a tin of tuna over a bed of steamed spinach or salad greens.

Midmorning or Midafternoon Mini-Meal

Mini-meals, or snacks, are to be eaten between meals, especially if many hours are going to pass before the next meal. These suggestions are also interchangeable: They are good between breakfast and lunch as well as between lunch and dinner.

- *Quick shake.* Same ingredients as the breakfast shake.
- *Protein bar.*
- *Low-fat cottage cheese and fruit.* Eight ounces/225 grams of low-fat cottage cheese and 4 ounces/115 grams of fresh fruit.
- *Protein mini-salad.* Four ounces/115 grams of sliced turkey, roast chicken, or lean roast beef over sliced tomatoes and cucumbers. Drizzle with flaxseed or olive oil and vinegar.
- *Yogurt and fruit.* Look for low-fat yogurt that has the term

acidophilus or *live yogurt cultures* on the label. These are excellent for reducing harmful bacteria in the intestinal tract (which we'll talk more about in chapter 11). You can buy fruit-flavored yogurt already mixed or, better yet, choose plain yogurt, add 4 ounces/115 grams of fruit, and sweeten with a bit of honey or maple syrup.
- *Soup.* Soup is always a treat, especially on a cold winter afternoon. Homemade soup is best, of course, made with chicken or turkey, fresh vegetables, and beef or chicken broth. If you're buying tinned soup, be sure to check the sodium content. Commercially prepared soup can be loaded with salt.
- Two hard-boiled eggs.

Lunch and Dinner Suggestions

Lunch and dinner meals are basically the same. They should include a protein, vegetables, and possibly a carbohydrate. Avoid desserts if possible (or save them for a special occasion), but if you want something sweet, have fruit. Here are some lunch or dinner suggestions:

- *Turkey salad.* Shred 4 ounces/115 grams of turkey and sprinkle it over a salad of mixed greens, tomato, cucumbers, and radishes. Season to taste. Make dressing with flaxseed, olive, or sesame oil and balsamic vinegar.
- *Tofu stir-fry.* Sauté 4 ounces/115 grams tofu in olive oil with kale, onions, carrots, and pea pods (or any other vegetables to your liking).
- *Hamburger and sweet potato.* Make your own quarter-pounder (minus the bun and the special sauce) with 4 ounces/115 grams lean mince (or better yet, substitute turkey mince). Layer with lettuce, tomato, and onion slices. Serve with half a sweet potato, garnished with a little butter and nutmeg, as a side dish.

- *Protein-salad-veggie meal.* Start your meal with an appetizer salad of mixed greens, tomatoes, and cucumbers. Then have an entrée of a serving of any protein—fish, chicken, turkey, lean beef—with steamed or grilled vegetables.
- *Salade nicoise.* Serve one hard-boiled egg, chunks of tuna, salad greens, tomato, and cucumbers with a dressing of oil and balsamic vinegar.

Bedtime Snack

If you feel you need something before you go to sleep, have some yogurt with 4 ounces/115 grams of fresh fruit. Or have some plain protein—4 ounces/115 grams of turkey is perfect for any metabolic type. It contains tryptophan, an amino acid that is known to have a sedating effect.

Suggestions for Eating Out

Staying on a food plan would be relatively easy if we stayed at home and cooked all our meals, but we don't. We're social creatures, and we sometimes meet friends for lunch or dinner. We celebrate occasions large and small by going out for a special treat. We are busy, busy, busy, and part of being so busy means we eat out or order in frequently. If you want to consider an occasional meal out "recreational eating," enjoy yourself. Order what you want, and have a pudding if you like. Then return to your metabolically correct food plan with your next meal.

However, there are ways to stay on the food plan and eat out at the same time. Here are some suggestions:

- *Chinese restaurant.* Many Chinese restaurants now offer "heart healthy" or "special diet" meals. Order steamed chicken, tofu, or shrimp with broccoli, green beans, pea pods, or mixed vegetables. Ask for the sauce on the side,

and use it sparingly. Eat only one-third to one-half the amount of rice served.
- *Italian restaurant.* Order chicken or fish, baked or broiled. When you order, ask how the dish will be prepared. You don't want anything smothered in butter or oil. Begin the meal with a Caesar salad (leave out the croûtons), and fill up on vegetables. Pass on the bread and the pasta. If you choose to have pasta, eat about one-third of what they serve you, and have it with tomato sauce rather than any type of cream sauce.
- *Mexican restaurant.* Order a chicken burrito with a wheat tortilla. Skip the guacamole and the sour cream, and instead ask for extra chicken and salsa. If the burrito is huge, as they are in most Mexican restaurants, cut it in two and take the other half home for another meal.
- *Fast-food chain.* Many fast-food restaurants are now offering salad choices, often with dressing in a side packet. If no salad is available, have a hamburger or cheeseburger with the lettuce, tomato, and onion, but without the bun.

AND DON'T FORGET TO EXERCISE

Yes, you do have to exercise. You may not want to—slow burners often dislike exercise—but you really should. Exercise not only will help you lose weight, but it is vital to your overall good health. It helps regulate appetite and facilitate digestion. It helps control insulin flow. It works to increase circulation and the intake of oxygen. In an article titled "How Exercise Works" (*Self*, 1993), author Royce Flippin states that it's not just burning calories that helps you lose weight, but "increases in blood flow and enzyme activity also improve the muscle fibers' ability to oxidize fats and carbohydrates carried in the blood—especially fats. That's one reason exercise is so effective for losing weight."

Flippin goes on to explain that "the ratio of 'good' (HDL) to 'bad' (LDL) cholesterol also improves with aerobic endurance—a major reason, along with improved circulation, why exercise helps ward off heart disease."

Exercise also helps you reduce your percentage of body fat. The body can be broken down into two types of weight: lean body weight, or LBW (muscles, bones, tendons, cartilage, and so on) and fat. When you figure out your body fat percentage, you can find out how much of your weight is LBW and how much is fat. For instance, a 100-pound (seven stone) woman with 20 percent body fat would consist of 80 pounds of LBW and 20 pounds of fat.

Body fat percentage can be measured in a number of ways, some complicated, some not so complicated. Most health club trainers and many doctors and health professionals use calipers. The "average" percentage of body fat for women is between 20 and 30 percent, depending on age (the percentage of body fat naturally increases as we get older). A woman with body fat above 40 percent is considered obese. For men, the average percentage of body fat ranges from 12 to 21 percent, depending on age. Obesity for men begins at about 30 percent. Many health professionals now believe that lowering the percentage of body fat is more important than lowering actual weight.

If you're a slow burner, you can stimulate your sluggish metabolism with aerobic exercise. Fitness expert Jonathan Bowden suggests that you will probably do best with relatively long and frequent workouts at a moderate intensity. Remember that aerobic exercises don't have to be done in a gym. Brisk walking, jogging, cross-country skiing, and bicycling are also beneficial aerobic exercises.

"The most important thing to remember is to start off slowly," says Bowden. "If you're not in shape, don't jump into a forty-five-minute aerobics class. You'll only be frustrated when you can't keep up. Set a realistic goal. If you can exercise intensely for only three minutes, allow yourself that success. Then increase your endurance a little bit every day. The point is to get yourself moving."

Phoebe L., age forty-two, came to see me about five months ago. Phoebe is five feet, five inches tall and weighed over 13 stone, with 32 percent body fat. She's an executive in the design field. She felt that her lack of energy was hurting her career. She'd been on medication for depression for about a year, and she suffered from chronic lower back pain. She had a long history of dieting and had been in and out of commercial diet programs for most of her adult life.

She had been trying to diet for a while, but she felt that her appetite was out of control. Any exercise caused her great fatigue. Her cholesterol level was high—about 140. She was depressed most of the time, and even though she knew that eating carbohydrates was making her fat, she said she felt better when she ate them. Phoebe's questionnaire showed she was a classic slow burner.

A typical day's diet for Phoebe was as follows:

Breakfast: two waffles with butter and maple syrup, two cups of coffee
Snack: apple
Lunch: baked potato covered with egg salad, roll with butter, fruit cup, and a cup of coffee
Dinner: salad with blue cheese dressing, chili over rice, and a brownie with vanilla ice cream.

After following the Balance program for slow burners, Phoebe's typical daily eating looks like this:

Breakfast: two eggs over easy on a bed of vegetables, one cup of herbal tea
Snack: designer shake
Lunch: small tin of tuna packed in water over salad greens and tomatoes with olive oil and balsamic vinegar, one pear
Snack: container of low-fat yogurt
Dinner: roast chicken with grilled vegetables

Phoebe has now dropped to 10 stone and decreased her percentage of body fat to 24. She's gone back to exercising and has much more endurance. She no longer drinks coffee, her back no longer hurts, and she has gone off antidepressants. (She does take St. John's wort, which I discuss in chapter 11). She's doing well in her career and is thinking of starting her own design firm.

9

ALL REVVED UP AND NO PLACE TO GO: SLOWING DOWN A FAST BURNER

WHAT'S THE HURRY?

Fast burners make up only about 20 percent of the population. If you have jumped right from taking the test in chapter 2 to this page because you are a fast burner, you might want to take a step that is somewhat unnatural for someone in your category. Slow down a minute. Go back and read the beginning of the previous chapter, specifically the information about the division of the nervous system and the description of the two parts and functions of the involuntary nervous system.

You will learn that the involuntary nervous system (which regulates functions over which we have no control, such as breathing, heart rate, and digestion) is divided into the sympathetic and parasympathetic nervous systems, and that fast burners are dominated by the sympathetic nervous system. The sympathetic nervous system controls the adrenal glands and the thyroid (see Figure 8.1). It is this system that is dominant in fast burners, and when it is overactive, it causes the release and burning of fuel too quickly, until ultimately the person burns out.

The adrenal glands, which are located just above the kidneys, secrete a number of hormones including adrenaline and cortisol. These two hormones work in concert to enable the body to deal with the demands of stress and energy. Both adrenaline and cortisol kick in when things get "exciting." In this case, the term *exciting* can have many connotations. You will get an adrenaline surge if you are being pursued by a rogue elephant, caught up in a strenuous argument, or asked to make a spontaneous presentation in front of a large group of people—anything that is considered stressful and provokes the fight-or-flight response. And the adrenaline surge can last a lot longer than the situation that made it occur in the first place. In fact, according to Mary Asterita, author of *The Physiology of Stress*, "the effect of these stress hormones can last about ten times as long as the sympathetic activity that caused them to be secreted because these hormones [adrenaline and cortisol] are removed from the circulation rather slowly."

It's easy to see what can happen when the adrenal glands are overactive. Instead of maintaining a neutral balance, the two adrenal hormones are constantly fighting with hormones of the parasympathetic nervous system, including insulin and glucagon. Adrenaline and cortisol are pushing you forward, while the parasympathetic hormones are elbowing their way in to keep you calm. This can result in frequent—and sometimes extreme—mood swings.

The thyroid gland, located on either side of the trachea, regulates the rates of metabolism and body growth. The excess production of thyroid hormones speeds up all body processes. It also interferes with the absorption of several essential minerals. Therefore, all nutrients in the body are depleted at a greater rate.

When both of these hormone producers are overactive, they cause your mineral reserves to become exhausted, thereby preventing you from obtaining optimum health and energy levels. Excessively high levels of cortisol, in fact, can burn critical amino acids necessary to muscle development.

A FAST BURNER IS . . .

Generalizations can be made about fast burners, as they were for slow burners, although here, too, individuality reigns. A majority of the characteristics listed will no doubt describe you, but there will be some that simply don't fit.

- Fast metabolizers are often described as type A personalities: overachievers who are often hyper and anxiety-ridden. They may also be described as *overarchers*, which means they have a greater reach than they can fulfill.
- Fast burners may suffer from hyperglycemia, or high blood sugar, a phenomenon in which too much cortisol is present. When this happens, you can be functioning in a state of temporary euphoria, or on a "sugar high." The problem is that when your blood sugar level drops, it often drops below normal, which can cause fatigue and irritability. This irritability often triggers the output of adrenaline and cortisol, which in turn helps to raise your blood sugar. Anxiety and irritability can become like a drug; you almost welcome these emotions because you may be more comfortable feeling speedy than sluggish.

- Fast burners often have addictive personalities. You may have obsessive-compulsive tendencies or develop substance abuse of drugs, alcohol, or food.
- Because the body is working overtime, fast burners may feel warm most of the time, have clammy palms and hands, and perspire easily. It doesn't take much physical activity to start the sweat pouring down. While the slow burners around you are closing their windows, you may be turning on the air conditioning.
- Fast burners often have bursts of intense mental activity, but long-term concentration can be difficult. That means you probably start a project (or two or three or four), get bored with it rather quickly, and go off to start something else.
- Fast burners may have trouble relaxing, or relaxation may have a different meaning for a fast burner than it does for a slow burner. You probably have difficulty taking naps. No sitting on the beach working on the perfect tan for you. If you take a vacation at all, it's probably to go mountain climbing or white-water rafting (and you take your mobile phone with you).
- One generalization that cannot be made, however, is that all fast burners are lean and mean. Although it might seem that burning all that fuel would keep you trim, it often has the opposite effect. When the adrenal is extremely overactive, it produces and overproduces cortisol, which can stimulate greater inflammation, water retention, and higher levels of sugar in the blood. The result is greater retention and storage of fat. The fast burner begins to put on weight, specifically in the abdominal region, which gives an apple-shaped body (see chapter 8 for the formula to help you determine your body shape).

- Fast burners may experience carbohydrate cravings, a phenomenon common to slow burners as well. For a fast burner, this happens because carbohydrates are metabolized so quickly that the body can't use them for energy. The stove is burning too hot, overheating the room and using up all the fuel. You look for more fuel in the form of carbohydrates. What happens next, however, is that your blood sugar shoots way up from the fast metabolizing of those carbohydrates, then falls way down again. So you feel the need for another carbohydrate energy boost. When you overload with carbohydrates, you increase your body's fat storage and become overweight.

Here are some generalized psychological and physiological traits of fast burners:

- Action orientation
- High motivation (quality of being driven)
- Quick anger
- Difficulty in falling asleep
- Dry eyes
- Elevated blood sugar levels
- Frequent exercising
- High blood pressure
- Impatience
- Impulsivity
- Jealousy
- Low calcium levels
- Low stress tolerance
- Profuse perspiration
- Sodium retention
- Ridged fingernails
- Excess worry

Following are some physical conditions and diseases fast burners are prone to:

- Acne
- Anemia
- Angina pectoris
- Anxiety
- Arteriosclerosis
- Bacterial infections
- Bronchitis
- Bursitis
- Conjunctivitis
- Diabetes (juvenile)
- Epilepsy
- Hodgkin's disease
- Hypertension
- Hyperthyroidism
- Leukemia
- Multiple sclerosis
- Parkinson's disease
- Rheumatoid arthritis (systemic, rather than localized)
- Ulcers

ON THE MENU

Figure 9.1, which outlines eight categories of foods, shows the foods that are preferable for a fast burner's diet. These are the foods that will help you slow down your runaway metabolism, decrease your burnout rate, and build up resistance to the diseases to which fast burners are susceptible. The general difference in diet between fast and slow burners slow is that fast burners can have heavier proteins, more fat, and a bit more of complex carbohydrates.

Figure 9.1

FOODS FOR FAST BURNERS

ANIMAL PROTEIN			VEGETABLE PROTEIN	VEGETABLES		FRUITS	GRAINS & GRAIN PRODUCTS	FATS & OILS	BEVERAGES	DESIGNER FOODS
Hoofed	Poultry	Seafood		Fibrous	Starchy					
Beef (lean)	Chicken	Anchovy	Tofu	Artichokes	Avocado	Apple	Brown rice	Olive oil	Herbal tea	Designer shakes
Lamb	Duck	Catfish	Tempeh	Asparagus	Beans	Apricot	Kasha	Sesame oil	Mineral water	Protein bars
Liver	Eggs	Clams		Aubergine	Legumes	Berries	Oatmeal	Canola oil	Vegetable juice	
Kidney	Goose	Cod		Bean sprouts	Potato	Cantaloupe melon	Quinoa	Flaxseed oil	Water	
Pork	Quail	Flounder		Beetroot	Squash	Cherry		Butter		
Veal	Turkey	Haddock		Broccoli	Sweet potato	Fig		Peanut butter		
Venison	Pheasant	Halibut		Brussels sprouts		Grapefruit		Almond butter		
		Herring		Cabbage		Honeydew melon		Cashew butter		
		Lobster		Carrots		Mango				
	Dairy	Mackerel		Cauliflower		Peach				
		Mussels		Celery		Pear				
	Cheese (all kinds)	Octopus		Cucumbers		Plum				
	Milk	Perch		Green beans		Water-melon				
	Yogurt	Salmon		Kale						
		Sardines		Lettuce						
		Scallops		Mushrooms						
		Scrod		Okra						
		Shrimp		Onions						
		Sole		Pea pods						
		Squid		Peppers						
		Swordfish		Spinach						
		Trout		Tomatoes						
		Tuna		Watercress						
		Turbot								

The food plan contains eight major categories:

1. Animal protein: hoofed animals, poultry, and seafood
2. Vegetable protein: soy products like tofu and tempeh
3. Vegetables: fibrous and starchy
4. Fruits
5. Grains and grain products
6. Fats and oils
7. Beverages
8. Designer foods

Animal Protein: Hoofed Animals, Poultry, and Seafood

In the last chapter, we established that all metabolic types (which means all human beings) need protein in their diets. While the lighter proteins—chicken and turkey, and fish such as flounder, sole, scrod, haddock, turbot, and perch—are fine for you if you're a fast burner, you can also add in some denser proteins. These are proteins higher in a substance called purine. Slow burners produce greater amounts of purines within their cells than do fast burners. Purines are found in red meat; wild game meat; and organ meats such as kidney, heart, liver, and sweetbreads. They are also found in cold-water and deep-ocean fish, including anchovies, herring, tuna, salmon, halibut, and sardines; these are the types of heart-healthy fish you should have at least once a week. These proteins can be broiled, boiled, roasted, baked, or grilled. Frying is the least desirable method of cooking.

If you're a fast burner, you can have more servings of dairy (three to four per week) than your slow-burning counterparts, because the calcium and fat in dairy will help slow your metabolism down. You can choose full-fat milk, cheeses, and yogurt.

Vegetarian Protein: Soy Products like Tofu and Tempeh

Tofu, tempeh, and other soy products are good choices for all metabolic types. Keep in mind that if you are using soy products as your only source of protein, you must eat portions large enough to equal the amount of animal protein you need. Even if you are a vegetarian, you should try to add in one or more fish meals and/or some eggs and cheese each week.

Vegetables: Fibrous and Starchy

The importance of eating your vegetables should not be underestimated. Fast burners do especially well with vegetables that are high in calcium and in vitamin A, including broccoli, cabbage, kale, and okra. Vegetables that are high in purine, including tomatoes, asparagus, artichokes, mushrooms, cauliflower, and spinach, also are beneficial to fast burners.

There is one caveat about high-purine foods, however. Some people are sensitive to purine and do not tolerate it well. In addition, purine is not good for people who suffer from gout. If you are a fast burner but are in either of the last two categories, reduce or eliminate purine-rich foods from your diet.

You should include at least four servings of fibrous vegetables a day (4 ounces/115 grams cooked or 8 ounces/225 grams raw is considered one serving). In fact, you may have as many servings of these vegetables as you like; however, consumption of starchy vegetables should be limited.

The main difference in food recommendations for fast and slow burners is the higher amount of purine-rich proteins recommended for fast burners. In addition, a fast burner may benefit from a complex carbohydrate breakfast (oatmeal, a baked potato, a sweet potato, or cooked rice cereal), along with a smaller amount of protein. Fast burners may consider having as many as four breakfast meals a week that contain complex carbohydrates.

Fruits

If you are a fast burner, you will probably do better if you limit the amount of fruit you have to two servings per day. The fruits usually recommended for fast burners are apples, pears, all types of berries, apricots, and melons. The stimulating effects of fruit can be cut somewhat if the fruit is eaten with a fat or protein, such as yogurt or cheese. Citrus fruits and bananas should be avoided by fast burners since both are loaded with potassium, a mineral that fast burners already have in relatively high levels. Potassium speeds up metabolism, which is not beneficial to fast burners.

Grains and Grain Products

Starchy carbohydrates should be limited, if not avoided altogether. That includes breads, rolls or baps, muffins, pastas, cold cereals, cakes and biscuits. Instead of eating these more "provocative" carbohydrates, choose basmati rice, cooked kasha, or quinoa. If you are going to have bread, try a multigrain variety.

Fats and Oils

Since fats tend to slow metabolism down, fast burners can add more fat into their diet than slow burners can. That means using about three tablespoons per day. If you have no problems tolerating dairy, you can choose greater amounts of calcium-bearing foods such as yogurt, cream, and cheeses. This also means choosing fattier dairy products, including full-fat milk, cheese, and yogurt. The choices of healthy fats for cooking and for salads are the same as they are for slow and mixed burners: flaxseed or sesame oil for salads, and olive or canola oil for cooking. You can also use butter to cook with or to sprinkle on vegetables, and you can include avocado, cream cheese, and nuts in your diet. (Be careful about the nuts; when nuts are treated as a snack food, it can be difficult to stop at just a few.) You can also add some nut butters to your diet, like almond butter and sunflower seed butter.

Beverages

The recommendations for slow burners apply here as well. *Drink at least eight glasses of water a day.* Choose from tap water, filtered water, and plain or flavored mineral water. A glass or two a day of vegetable juice can be a tasty addition to your liquid intake, but beware the sodium! You can get low- or no-sodium versions of vegetable juice and add your own salt if you feel you need it. In general, fast oxidizers should limit their intake of salt or sodium because it tends to aggravate the already overstimulated adrenal gland.

If you're a fast burner, you should stay away from fruit juice. Fruit is stimulating enough, but when you eliminate the fiber and drink it in its pure form, it's like pouring petrol on a fire. It will immediately raise your blood sugar level and speed up your metabolism, and then it will wear off just as quickly, leaving you down in the dumps and craving something sweet.

Like slow burners, you should limit your intake of soft drinks. Both diet and regular sodas contain phosphoric acid, which interferes with the absorption of calcium. Fast burners already have lower levels of calcium, so they should not put anything in the way of getting the amounts needed.

Designer Foods: Shakes and Power Bars

The information included in chapter 8, for slow burners, applies also to fast burners. Shake mixes and power bars are readily available in most health food stores.

STRUCTURING YOUR DAY

Fast burners often eat all day long. Because your fuel is burned up so quickly, you always seem to be in need of more. If you're a fast burner, you may find yourself exceedingly hungry between meals, and you may even experience dizziness or feel light-headed. Therefore, it's important to keep up your fuel supply by including mini-meals in between your regular meals. Remember that the following meal suggestions are interchangeable: Breakfasts, lunches, and dinners all have equal value, and snacks can be eaten at any time during the day. You can also check out the meal suggestions for slow burners. Any of those are appropriate for fast burners as well. The only difference is that whole eggs can be substituted for egg whites, and whole-fat dairy products can be substituted for low-fat versions.

Breakfast Suggestions

No matter what metabolic type you are, your breakfast should contain protein to give your day the proper energy foundation. If you enjoy fruit in the morning, have one-quarter of a melon (honeydew, cantaloupe, galia) or 4 ounces/115 grams of a variety of berries (use fresh fruit, not tinned or frozen, whenever possible). Here are some breakfast options a fast burner might consider:

- *The quick shake.* This energy-boosting shake is only slightly different from the one suggested for slow burners. If you're a fast burner, use two scoops of Ultra Clear and one scoop of Designer Protein. Mix in the blender with 6–8 fluid ounces/175–225ml of water. Add in one tablespoon of flaxseed oil. You can also add 4 ounces/115 grams of papaya, strawberries, blueberries, or raspberries.
- *The three-egg vegetable omelet.* You can use three whole eggs or two whole eggs and the whites of one more (cooked

with one-half to one tablespoon of olive oil). Add 2 ounces/50 grams each of some of your favorite vegetables, like mushrooms, broccoli, peppers, and onions.
- *The cheese omelet.* Same as the three-egg variety, with the addition of 2 ounces/50 grams of any type of cheese.
- *Oatmeal and eggs.* If you want a heartier breakfast, have 8 ounces/225 grams oatmeal (sweetened with a touch of honey or maple syrup or a handful of raisins) and two poached or hard-boiled eggs.
- *Steak and eggs.* Use 2–3 ounces/50–85 grams of lean beef with two whole eggs. It can be served with half a potato.
- *Sausage and eggs.* Use two lean pork sausages and scrambled eggs cooked in olive oil.
- *Peanut, almond, or cashew butter and apples.* Spread one tablespoon of freshly ground nut butter on apple slices (you can grind peanut butter yourself in some health food stores).

Midmorning or Midafternoon Mini-Meal

Mini-meal, or snack, suggestions are to be eaten between meals, especially when many hours are going to pass before you get to eat your lunch or dinner. These suggestions are also interchangeable: good between breakfast and lunch as well as between lunch and dinner.

- *Quick shake.* Same ingredients as the breakfast shake.
- *Protein bar.*
- *Cottage cheese and fruit.* Eight ounces/225 grams of cottage cheese and 4 ounces/115 grams of fresh fruit.
- *Yogurt and fruit.* Whether you choose a low-fat or full-fat version of yogurt, be sure to choose a brand that has the term *acidophilus* or *live yogurt cultures* on the label. You can

buy fruit-flavored yogurt already mixed or, better yet, choose plain yogurt, add 4 ounces/115 grams of fruit, and sweeten with a bit of honey or maple syrup.

Lunch and Dinner Suggestions

Lunch and dinner meals are basically the same. They should include a protein, vegetables, and possibly a carbohydrate. Avoid puddings if possible, but if you want something sweet, have fruit. Here are some lunch or dinner suggestions:

- *Chef salad.* Shred 4 ounces/115 grams of turkey, 4 ounces/115 grams of lean roast beef, and 2 ounces/50 grams of Swiss cheese, and sprinkle them over a salad of mixed greens, tomato, cucumbers, and radishes. Season to taste. Make dressing with flaxseed, olive, or sesame oil, and balsamic vinegar.
- *Chicken Caesar salad.* Serve sliced baked or broiled chicken over a bed of lettuce with a small portion of classic Caesar dressing. Sprinkle freely with Parmesan cheese.
- *Salmon salad.* Mix 4 ounces/115 grams or a tin of salmon with chopped carrots, chopped salad onions, and sprouts. Add olive oil and balsamic vinegar or a tablespoon of low-fat mayonnaise.
- *Buckwheat pasta and shrimp.* Buckwheat, also known as kasha, is not related to wheat and contains no gluten. Buckwheat pasta is sometimes called soba noodles. Follow cooking instructions on the package of pasta, add six shrimp and a few olives, and season to taste. Serve with a side dish of steamed or grilled vegetables.
- *Liver and onions.* Choose calves' liver or chicken livers. Bake, broil, or sauté with onions, peppers, and seasonings.

Bedtime Snack

If you feel you need to eat something before you go to sleep, have some yogurt with 4 ounces/115 grams of fresh fruit. Or have some plain protein: Four ounces/115 grams of turkey is perfect because it contains tryptophan, an amino acid that is known to have a sedating effect.

Suggestions for Eating Out

No one expects you to eat every meal at home. Allow yourself the occasional indulgent meal for your recreational eating, and then return to your regular eating routine with your next meal. Following are some suggestions for staying on the food plan and eating out at the same time:

- *Chinese restaurant.* Many Chinese restaurants now offer "heart healthy" or "special diet" meals. Order steamed chicken, tofu, shrimp, or beef with broccoli, green beans, pea pods, or mixed vegetables. Ask for the sauce on the side, and use about half of what you're given, along with one-half the amount of brown rice served.
- *Italian restaurant:* Order chicken, fish, or veal, baked or broiled. Begin the meal with a Caesar salad (leave out the croûtons) and fill up on vegetables. If you choose to have pasta, eat about one-half of what is served. You may have either cream sauce or tomato sauce.
- *Mexican restaurant.* Order a chicken burrito with a wheat tortilla, including guacamole and sour cream. Ask for extra chicken and salsa. Since the burritos served in most Mexican restaurants are huge, cut yours in two and take the other half home for another meal.
- *Fast-food chains.* Many fast-food restaurants are now offering salad choices, often with dressing in a side packet. If no salad is available, have a hamburger or cheeseburger with the lettuce, tomato, and onion, but without the bun.

AND DON'T FORGET TO EXERCISE

Years ago, nobody had to look for ways to exercise. It was part of the way people lived. They worked hard and walked long distances. Today, you have to find time in your busy life to jog in the park or get to the gym. Alternatively, if you have the space and the money, you can set up equipment at home. However you choose to do it, be sure you get your exercise. See chapter 8 for an explanation of exactly what exercise does for your body.

If you're a fast burner, you don't want to overstimulate your system with a lot of heavy aerobics. You're better off with exercise that burns fat and tones your body but at a slower rate, such as weight training, swimming, casual bike riding, and walking. As always, if you're out of shape, start very slowly and increase your pace gradually.

> Eileen R. is a forty-year-old vice president of a banking firm. She travels extensively for business and practically lives in hotels and airplanes. She is extremely driven and ambitious, and she told me she was tense all the time. Exercise made her feel better, but she could never find the time for it. She'd gained one and a half stone in the last four years. Her eating was extremely haphazard, and she sometimes went for long stretches without food.
>
> When she came to see me, she was taking no medications, but she said she was addicted to Diet Coke and drank at least eight to ten cans daily. A typical day's menu looked like this:
>
> 6:00 A.M.: Diet Coke, container of fat-free cottage cheese
> 10:00 A.M.: Diet Coke
> 11:30 A.M.: Diet Coke
> 1:00 P.M.: Twelve ounces/340 grams of fresh peas with one-half tin of tuna, Diet Coke
> 2:45 P.M.: Diet Coke
> 4:30 P.M.: Diet Coke

The Balance

    8:00 P.M.: Piece of chicken, vegetables, baked potato, Diet Coke
10:45 P.M.: Diet Coke

After beginning the Balance program for fast burners, her daily eating pattern looked like this:

   7:00 A.M.: Four ounces/115 grams of oatmeal with omelet made from three egg whites, glass of water
10:00 A.M.: Two yogurts, glass of water
12:00 noon: Salmon salad with tomatoes and cucumbers, olive oil and vinegar
  3:00 P.M.: Protein shake
  6:30 P.M.: Six ounces/170 grams of lamb with steamed vegetables, glass of water
10:45 P.M.: Four ounces/115 grams of sliced turkey breast

Eileen has lost one and a quarter stone so far, and she now weighs just over 9 stone. Her body fat is at 26 percent. She works out four times a week at home in the morning. When she travels, she stays at a hotel that has a gym. She is careful about planning her day so that she has all three meals, and she snacks whenever she can. She no longer drinks Diet Coke at all. She says she is more relaxed—and more productive—than she ever was.

10

THE MIXED BURNER: DON'T ROCK THE BOAT

MAINTAINING THE BALANCE

This is a short chapter. There aren't many mixed burners around. Theoretically, only 10 percent of the population fall into this category, and in reality, that figure is probably too high.

If you are a mixed burner, it means that you exhibit traits of both fast and slow burners. There are times where you are being pulled in the direction of a fast burner, and other times where your metabolism more highly resembles a slow burner. You are often teetering between the two. On the other hand, there are times when mixed burners are evenly balanced. That means that your sympathetic and parasympathetic nervous systems are doing exactly what they're supposed to be doing, in just the right proportions. Your body is experiencing the perfect balance of glandular activity and metabolic function.

If you are a mixed burner, you can consider yourself lucky. You are usually closer to being balanced than the other two types of burners. That means you have great choice in the foods you eat. You can enjoy and thrive on foods from both the fast and slow burner categories.

That doesn't mean, however, that you can eat whatever you want, whenever you want. The downside of being a mixed burner is that the balance you have is a precarious one. You can easily slide off in either direction. If you do not follow the guidelines of good eating, if you consume mass quantities of processed foods, if you drink many cups of coffee each day, you will suffer the consequences. Your health, weight, and emotional well-being are all affected by what you eat. Being a mixed burner isn't a free ride.

Outside influences are a factor as well. If you're going through a stressful period, your normally stable metabolism can easily get off kilter. The best way to minimize the damage is to continue to make smart, healthy food choices.

A MIXED BURNER IS . . .

As in the other two categories, there are some gross generalizations that can be made about mixed burners. Here are some psychological and physiological traits of mixed burners:

- Doesn't mind exercise when there is time to do it.
- Keeps emotions on an even keel.
- Falls asleep within a reasonable period of time.
- Handles stress well most of the time.
- Has a fair amount of ambition and drive.

The Balance 153

- Has a high pain tolerance.
- Likes a wide variety of foods.
- Needs extra sleep every once in a while.
- Occasionally gets angry.
- Occasionally has periods of fatigue.
- Seldom experiences between-meal hunger.
- Wakes up rested and gets started easily.

Here are some physical characteristics of mixed burners and some diseases they are prone to:

- Good digestion
- Infrequent asthma attacks
- Infrequent, short-duration colds
- Normal blood pressure
- Normal perspiration
- Occasional acne
- Occasional stomach ache
- Rarely, diabetes

MIX YOUR MENU

Figure 10.1 presents eight categories of foods. Any of the food choices in this chart are appropriate for you.

If you are a mixed burner, go back and read the last two chapters. There you'll find valuable information on each of the food categories, as well as some menu suggestions and tips for eating out. Choose those that appeal to you most, and keep a record of how you feel after you eat various foods. If you feel better when you follow the guidelines for a slow burner, perhaps you are leaning in that direction. If the fast burner menu feels better to you, stick with those choices. You are the only one who can truly judge which foods allow you to perform at your peak performance capacity.

Figure 10.1

FOODS FOR MIXED BURNERS

ANIMAL PROTEIN			VEGETABLE PROTEIN	VEGETABLES		FRUITS	GRAINS & GRAIN PRODUCTS	FATS & OILS	BEVERAGES	DESIGNER FOODS
Hoofed	Poultry	Seafood		Fibrous	Starchy					
Beef (lean)	Chicken	Anchovy	Tofu	Artichokes	Avocado	Apple	Brown rice	Olive oil	Herbal tea	Designer shakes
Lamb	Duck	Catfish	Tempeh	Asparagus	Beans	Apricot	Corn	Sesame oil	Mineral water	Protein bars
Liver	Eggs	Clams		Aubergine	Legumes	Banana	Couscous	Canola oil	Vegetable juice	
Kidney	Goose	Cod		Bean sprouts	Potato	Berries	Kasha	Flaxseed oil	Water	
Pork	Quail	Flounder		Beetroot	Squash	Cantalope melon	Oatmeal	Butter		
Veal	Turkey	Haddock		Broccoli		Cherry	Quinoa	Peanut butter		
Venison	Pheasant	Halibut		Brussels sprouts		Fig		Almond butter		
		Herring		Cabbage		Grapefruit		Cashew butter		
Dairy		Lobster		Carrots		Grape				
		Mackerel		Cauliflower		Honeydew melon				
		Mussels		Celery		Mango				
Cheese (all kinds)		Octopus		Cucumbers		Orange				
Milk		Perch		Green beans		Papaya				
Yogurt (all kinds)		Salmon		Kale		Peach				
		Sardines		Lettuce		Pear				
		Scallops		Mushrooms		Pineapple				
		Scrod		Okra		Plum				
		Shrimp		Onions		Watermelon				
		Sole		Pea pods						
		Squid		Peppers						
		Swordfish		Spinach						
		Trout		Tomatoes						
		Tuna		Watercress						
		Turbot								

MIX YOUR EXERCISE

The same concept of experimentation that you apply to choosing your foods should go into choosing your exercise. You can mix and match your exercises, alternating between aerobics and resistance training. There may be times when you feel the need to speed your system up; that's when aerobics will be the best choice. If you want to slow yourself down, try a period of weight training. Choose activities you enjoy so that you are more likely to continue being active.

11

HOW TO LIVE FOREVER: THE NEW SCIENCE OF HEALTH

THE QUEST TO LIVE FOREVER

In a perfect world, we would all live forever, or at least for a very long time. The world would be crowded, of course, but we'd figure out a way to deal with that. We wouldn't live in a world of the invalid elderly either. People would live long, healthy lives well into their 120s, 130s, or 140s.

Sounds impossible? It wasn't so many years ago that humans couldn't imagine anyone living past the age of forty. Life was too hard, there were too many incurable diseases, there was so much that was still to be discovered. Life is still hard today; there are still a number of incurable diseases; and there is still much to be discovered. The difference is that in the recent past years separated the exciting discoveries that helped extend life expectancy. Now these discoveries are separated by days.

Every day you can turn on the television, read the newspaper, or surf the web and find another amazing announcement. Scientists have uncovered the gene mutation that causes another disease. They have discovered that it's slow damage to the teeny tiny tips of our chromosomes that makes us age, and as soon as they find the way to stop that from happening, we'll live to be as old as Methuselah. In addition, every day some scientist seems to discover *the* definitive hormone that makes us hungry, makes us fat, makes us unable to control our runaway appetites. Or at least researchers have discovered what makes *rats* hungry. Give them another five or ten or fifteen years, and they'll figure out how it works in humans. In another ten years or so, they'll figure out the cure for the common cold, and on and on.

It's overwhelming. We are learning more and more about our bodies, how they work (and why they sometimes don't work very well), and what we can do to help them work more efficiently. One of the areas in which scientists, doctors, and nutritionists have made great strides is in how taking supplements—vitamins, minerals, and herbs—can help us live longer, healthier lives. Today, many of us use some form of supplementation. For many, this has changed from taking one multivitamin a day to taking multiple supplements with every meal. Even the most conservative members of the medical community are starting to acknowledge the benefits of using supplements, along with proper nutrition and exercise, as part of an overall plan for healthy living.

In this chapter, I attempt to clear up some of the confusion about supplements, explaining how they work and what purposes they serve. The supplement recommendations in this chapter apply no matter what metabolic type you are. Anyone can run into the kinds of problems supplements are designed to fix. For instance, even though you are a fast burner, you may be experiencing fatigue and can benefit from supplements that will help get you back in balance. We're going to talk about how some supplements can booster your general health, while others are most beneficial for dealing with particular problems and illnesses. But before we get to that, we have to talk about the reasons we need supplements in the first place.

THE TOXIC TIME BOMB

Remember the fish tank you had when you were a kid? You loved having it, but it took work to keep the fish alive. You had to have a filter, and the filter had to be taken out and cleaned periodically. And then there were the times you had to find your little white net, scoop out the fish, place them temporarily into a plastic bag full of water, and scrub the gunk off the sides of the tank. If you neglected these steps, it was fatal for the fish.

Our bodies have several different filtering systems, including the following:

- *Intestines.* In their healthy state, the intestines help get rid of toxins through regular bowel movements, by eliminating unhealthy microorganisms, and by providing a strong barrier against leakage into the blood system.
- *Liver.* The liver filters out and transforms toxins that have entered the bloodstream into harmless substances that can be excreted in the urine.

- *Kidney.* The kidney's main purpose is to provide the major escape route for toxins, through the urine.
- *Skin.* We sweat through the pores in our skin. Sweat is an excellent system for releasing many of the toxins in the body, which is one of the reasons we smell so bad after a good sweaty workout.
- *Fat.* Although fat is not a filtering system per se, the reduction of fat helps eliminate toxins. Excess toxins often deposit themselves in fat cells, where they tend to stay, and the only way to get rid of those toxins is to get rid of the excess fat—in other words, lose weight.

We can't take these filtering systems out every so often, like fish tank filters, and give them a good cleaning. Therefore, we have to find ways of cleaning out the system from within. If we don't, the result can prove fatal for us as well; it is what I call the "toxic time bomb."

WHAT ARE TOXINS?

Toxins are poisonous materials. They can come from the air we breathe, the food we eat, and the water we drink. They come from pesticides and smog and bus fumes and industrial chemicals. They are in our systems as the residue of drugs—legal and illegal—we have taken over the years. They are in the alcohol we drink and in the cigars and cigarettes we smoke (not to mention the tobacco we chew). They enter the body along with the artificial colorings, flavorings, and preservatives in our food supply.

We even produce our own toxins. Our intestinal tract houses many kinds of bacteria, some healthy and some unhealthy. When there are too many unhealthy bacteria, they release toxic by-products into our system, which contribute to many diseases and general feelings of ill health.

Although the body has been designed with several built-in filtration systems, these systems cannot always handle the overload of today's toxic environments. The consequences of this toxic overload are wide ranging. They include:

- Allergies
- Alzheimer's disease
- Bad breath
- Bowel problems
- Cardiovascular problems
- Depression
- Fatigue
- Gastrointestinal tract irregularities
- Headache
- Irritability
- Muscle and joint pain
- Parkinson's disease
- PMS

DETOXIFICATION: STARTING WITH A CLEAN SLATE

If toxins are so harmful to our systems, we need to know how to get rid of them. There are various methods we can use to detoxify, or cleanse our systems.

Nutrition

What you eat greatly affects how toxic you are. You wouldn't feed your pet fish sweets, cakes, and refined wheat products, would you? Can you imagine what these unnatural substances would do to their systems? In fact, these foods wreak similar havoc with our systems. When toxins leak through an unhealthy intestine and flow to the liver, the liver begins its own two-part process of detoxification.

In phase 1, a "superfamily" of enzymes called the cytochrome P450 system transforms the toxins into what are called *metabolites*. In phase 2, these metabolites are further transformed so that they can be eliminated in the urine or feces. Sometimes, however, the transformation is incomplete; the metabolites get stuck in their phase 1 form and remain toxic. This is why you sometimes feel worse during the detoxification process; until it's complete, you may be producing even more toxins than before. Not only that, the metabolites that are formed then produce free radicals (which I talked about in chapter 5 and will talk about more a little later). These free radicals are what do us harm.

What does nutrition have to do with this? Not too long ago, it was thought that water and juice fasts were effective in clearing toxins out of the body. But a study published in the *Annual Review of Nutrition* in 1991 showed that fasting actually decreases protection against free radicals. It also showed that efficient functioning of the cytochrome P450 system requires adequate dietary protein; furthermore, it appears that a high carbohydrate intake reduces the ability of the P450 enzymes to work effectively. The best way to bolster your natural detoxification system, therefore, is to follow the Balance program, with its relatively high-protein, low-carbohydrate foods.

Exercise

One of the major ways to get rid of toxins is by sweating. Any type of exercise that makes you sweat, whether aerobics or weight training, is good for you. In an article in the *Journal of Holistic Medicine*, Drs. Elmer M. Cranston and James P. Frackleton wrote, "Proper oxygenation enhances defenses against free radicals. Aerobic exercise stimulates blood flow and improves oxygen utilization, resulting in adequate oxygenation to remote capillary beds. ... Oxygen acts as a free radical scavenger during exercise and reduces free radical pathology." If you're just starting an exercise program, it's a good idea to join a fitness club and work with a trainer to design a program for you. If you can't do that, read *Smart Exercise* by Covert Bailey as a guide.

Steam and Sauna

Even more effective than exercise in causing detoxification through sweat are steam baths and saunas. I experienced an effective program a few years ago when I joined the local YMCA. For three weeks, I went to the gym every morning and alternated the steam bath and sauna for an hour. After the first week, I felt awful. Halfway through the second week, I was sitting in the sauna by myself when I detected the odor of stale tobacco. I wondered who had been smoking in the sauna. To my surprise, I realized the odor was coming from my body, and I haven't smoked in fifteen years! After that, I began to feel better than I had for many years.

Start off by sitting in the steam or sauna for short periods of time—five or ten minutes. Build up to half an hour, taking a break every ten or fifteen minutes.

Ultra Clear

Ultra Clear is a rice powder shake developed by Jeffrey Bland of the Metagenics company, made from a patented metabolic formula specially designed to detoxify the system. It can be used on a daily basis as part of your protein shake breakfast or snack. If you want a stronger detoxification program, you can follow a modified Ultra Clear program once a week or once a month. Any metabolic type can follow this plan.

On arising, have an Ultra Clear shake, then have another midmorning. For lunch, have a cup of basmati rice with vegetables such as broccoli, peas, asparagus, pea pods, cabbage, cauliflower, or green beans. Midday, have another shake along with a pear. For dinner, have another cup of rice with vegetables with a little olive oil. You can have another shake and another piece of fruit before bedtime. This one-day program gives the system a rest from digesting difficult foods and allows the body to cleanse and detoxify itself. The next day, go back to the food plan that is appropriate for your metabolic type.

You should always check with a health care professional before embarking on any extensive detoxification program. Although nothing suggested here should prove harmful, it's best to be sure that the program you choose is right for you.

DAMAGE CONTROL: ANTIOXIDANTS AND LONGEVITY

The reason the toxins that come from both inside and outside the body are so harmful is that they produce free radicals. As discussed in chapter 5, a free radical is an oxygen molecule with an odd number of electrons in the outer ring of one of its atoms. Free radicals are produced by natural chemical reactions in the body and are necessary for health. However, stress—chemical stress, emotional stress, physical trauma, and infection—creates an overproduction of free radicals.

Free radicals are destructive because they try to "steal" electrons from healthy cells. There are billions of cells in the body, and we create millions more every day. When there is excess free radical activity in the body, we destroy more cells than we can create. The longer the destruction of cells continues, the greater the damage to our health.

As we age, and when we succumb to disease, our cells are being overrun by free radicals. You can see free radical damage on the skin. Free radicals cause skin cells to collapse and harden; this causes the skin to sag, resulting in wrinkles. Another visible sign of free radical damage is age spots. When you see brown spots on your hands or face as you get older, what you're seeing is the spoilage, or oxidation, of your own fat. That kind of oxidative damage is also occurring internally to your lungs, your liver, your heart, and your brain.

Our bodies produce natural free-radical fighters called *antioxidants*. As Steven Fowkes explained in the April 15, 1996, issue of *Smart Drug News*, "antioxidants function by offering easy electron targets for free radicals. In absorbing a free radical, antioxidants 'trap' (de-energize or stabilize) the lone free radical electron and make it stable enough to be transported to an enzyme which combines two stabilized free radicals together to neutralize both."

If you want to live a longer, healthier life, the best way to do it is to reduce the amount of free radical damage in your body. One of the best ways to remove free radical activity is to relieve yourself of stress. This is not always practical, however; there are some forms of stress, such as noise and industrial pollution, that we can't easily avoid. And life periodically puts us in stressful situations that we have to endure.

The next best way to reduce free radical damage is to bolster the power of the natural antioxidants found in our body, such as vitamin C, vitamin E, and beta-carotene. Your diet should include foods rich in these nutrients, including broccoli, cabbage, cauliflower, kale, spinach, brussels sprouts, tomato, courgettes, winter squash, strawberries, oranges, and grapefruit. Unfortunately, it may be difficult to eat enough of these fruits and vegetables to keep up with free radical damage. Fortunately, we now have a wide variety of powerful antioxidant supplements available. At the end of this book, you will find a glossary that explains the properties and functions of many of those supplements. Here are the ones I recommend for bringing the body back into free-radical balance:

Supplement	Amount per day
Vitamin C	1000 mg
Vitamin E	400 IU
Selenium	100 micrograms
Glutathione	300 mg
Coenzyme Q-10	30 mg
DMG	125 mg
Grape seed extract	60 mg
Ginkgo biloba	500 mg

There are also general antioxidant formulas, sold by several different manufacturers, in which these ingredients have been put together in one megasupplement. I recommend Life Extension Mix by the Life Extension Foundation.

SUPPLEMENT SUGGESTIONS: CHART AND GLOSSARY

Besides antioxidants, there are many other kinds of supplements that can help to improve your health. Because sorting out these supplements can be confusing, I have divided the best-known ones into twelve categories. Using Figures 11.1 and 11.2, you can choose the category you're interested in enhancing and find a list of supplements that apply. If you're not sure what a particular supplement is or does, look it up in the glossary.

Most vitamins and other supplements do not cause any health problems themselves. However, excessive use of individual products can be unhealthy; you should always consult with your health care provider or nutritionist before taking a new supplement, especially if you are taking prescriptions or other over-the-counter medications. If you experience any side effects from a supplement, stop taking it immediately. However, be realistic about what's causing these side effects. A client of mine once told me she had

FIGURE 11.1

IMMUNITY/RISK PREVENTION	ANTI-AGING	ENERGY ENHANCERS
Acidophilus	Bilberry	Creatine monohydrate
Carotenoids	DHEA	DMG
DHA (not to be confused with DHEA)	Ginkgo biloba	HMB
Echinacea	IP-6/Inositol	l-tyrosine
Garlic	Licopene	NADH
Goldenseal	Lutein	
Grapefruit seed oil	Melatonin	
Green tea extract	Vitamin E	
Olive leaf extract		
Omega-3, omega-6		
Saw palmetto		
Selenium		
Soya isoflavonoids		
St. John's Wort		
Vitamin C		
Whey peptides		

MOOD ENHANCERS	CARDIOVASCULAR HEALTH	ANTIOXIDANTS
Light therapy	Coenzyme Q-10	Alpha lipoic acid
l-tyrosine	DMG	Coenzyme Q10
NADH	Folic acid	DMG
Negative ionizers	Garlic	Ginkgo biloba
St. John's Wort	Magnesium	Glutathione
SAM	NADH	NAC
	Omega-3, omega-6	Selenium
	Pantethine	Vitamin C
	Vitamin E	Vitamin E
	Vitamin B12	Huprizine A
		Grape seed extract

terrible heart palpitations in reaction to a supplement I'd suggested to her. I asked her to tell me what happened. "Well," she said, "it was the day we were trying to decide whether or not to take the company into bankruptcy. We had a meeting in the morning. I didn't have time for breakfast, so I took the supplement with

FIGURE 11.2

SMART NUTRIENTS/ BRAIN BOOSTERS	WEIGHT MANAGEMENT/ METABOLIC ENHANCERS	CRAVING CONTROL
Acetyl-L-Carnitine CDP/Choline DMAE Ginkgo biloba Pregnenolone St. John's Wort	Burn Fat by Equinox* Designer Protein by NEXT* Energenics by Metagenics* Fiberfood by Life Extension Foundation* HEAT by Metoform* MCT Oil by Perillo* Pyruvate Sea Klenz by Wachters*	Chromium Glutamine St. John's Wort Hydroxycitrate

HORMONES & HORMONE BALANCERS	DETOXIFIERS	MUSCLE BUILDERS
Calcium Dong quai Gota kola Vitamin B6 For Women Only by Allergy Research* DHEA Bio-PMT by Thorne Research* Soy isoflavones Magnesium citrate Omega-3, omega-6 P5P by Douglas Laboratories*	Dandelion Glutathione Milk thistle NAC Ultra Clear by Metagenics*	Creatine monohydrate Glutamine HMB by E.A.S.* Whey peptides

*Proprietary Formula/Brand Name

two cups of coffee. Then I got these terrible heart palpitations." It became obvious to me that the palpitations had been caused not by the supplement, but by the fact that she took it with coffee and on an empty stomach on a day when she was undergoing extreme stress. Always take supplements with food unless specifically told otherwise, and be aware of unusual influences (such as stress or anxiety) that may be "causing" the side effect.

It took me a while to convince this woman that the palpitations and the supplement may not have had a direct cause-and-effect relationship. I asked her to take a few days off and then to try the supplement again the following week, when things had calmed down. She had no complaints the second time around.

PRESCRIPTIONS FOR SPECIAL PROBLEMS

When you follow the Balance program and eat according to what's best for your metabolic type, you may find that some of the illnesses and ailments to which you are usually prone will begin to disappear. However, metabolic balance doesn't happen overnight. Your body has the results of many years of being off kilter to counteract. Therefore, you may want to help your body adjust by taking supplements that can help straighten out a metabolic imbalance.

As you read the lists of recommended supplements, remember that you don't have to take all of them to get a positive effect. After discussing the subject with a health professional, try taking one or two and see what happens. Make yourself a scientific experiment, just as you do with the foods you eat. Keep trying various combinations of supplements until you find the ones that work best for you.

In chapter 6, I discussed how supplementation can help relieve the symptoms of PMS and the menopause. In this chapter, I look at five other problems that require special solutions. Once again, you can find descriptions of all recommended supplements in the glossary in Appendix A.

Weight Management Products and Metabolism Enhancers

Most of the supplements recommended for losing weight are made up of "thermogenic agents." *Thermogenics* is a term that refers to anything that stimulates the burning of fat. Both fast and slow burners can use weight management products and metabolism enhancers. There are so many weight loss products on the market that it's difficult to tell which are truly beneficial and which are scams. To determine which is which you have to educate yourself, for example by reading reputable publications. Do some research in your local library or at a healthfood store to determine which publications keep track of new product development and give unbiased analyses of each product they review.

Following are some supplements you can take to help you reach your weight loss goals, along with recommended dosages. If you want to take higher dosages, consult manufacturers' recommendations and/or your health care practitioner.

Supplement	Amount per day
Energenics by Metagenics*	2 tablets
MCT Oil by Perillo*	1000 mg
Burn Fat by Equinox*	1000 mg
Designer Protein by NEXT*	1–2 shakes
HEAT by Metoform*	Follow manufacturer's recommendations
Fiberfood Powder by Life Extension Foundation*	3–4 times a week
Sea Klenz by Wachter	1–2 tablespoons
Pyruvate	Follow manufacturer's recommendations
Branched chain amino acids	1000 mg
CLA oil	Follow manufacturer's recommendations

*Proprietary formula/brand name

Compromised Immune System

How many colds did you get last year? How many times were you "under the weather" with the flu? If you were out of commission more than two or three times, it may be because your immune system (your body's natural ability to fight off disease and infection) is weak. If you work or live in close proximity to others—and who doesn't?—you're constantly exposed to germs, bacteria, and viruses that are easily passed from one person to another. Many people find themselves chronically weakened by what seems to be one continuous cold or flu. This can be extremely debilitating.

Following are the supplements I recommend to begin to bolster a weakened immune system, along with recommended dosages:

Supplement	Amount per day
Alive & Well by Nutricology* (olive leaf extract)	100 mg
Vitamin C	At least 1000 mg
DHA (not to be confused with DHEA)	500 mg
St. John's Wort	At least 300 mg
Garlic	500 mg
Whey peptide shake	3–4 times a week

*Proprietary formula/brand name

Fatigue

Fatigue is one of the most common complaints I hear from clients when they first come to see me. Their energy levels are low, and they are tired all the time. Of course, most people lead extremely busy lives, but that's not the only explanation for their fatigue. Usually it's due to poor diet and metabolic imbalance.

The issue of energy and fatigue is a complex one, given that there are so many factors that come into play. First of all, everyone has a different perception of what it means to be a vital individual. Some people are used to high energy levels, and anything below that level feels inadequate. Other people are normally low key and may feel that they're "supposed" to feel differently. What you want is to be able to get a good night's sleep and wake up in the morning feeling rested. You want to have enough energy to take you through the day with optimum brain function. You want to have adequate energy at the end of the work week so that you don't simply collapse Friday evening and have to sleep all weekend.

You can improve your energy level greatly by eating the foods that are metabolically correct for you and, especially, by eliminating foods—excess carbohydrates, refined flour and sugar—that contribute to exhaustion. In addition, you can choose from the following supplements that are intended to enhance energy levels. Start with one, and see how you feel. If it doesn't suit you, try another one. Don't take all of them at once.

Supplement	Amount per day
NADH	2.5 mg (on rising)
DMG	125 mg, 2 times
Acetyl-L-carnitine	500–1000 mg
Creatine monohydrate	1–3 grams
Energenics by Metagenics*	1–2 tablets
Whey peptide shake	3–4 times a week
Choline Cocktail by Twin Labs*	follow manufacturer's recommendations

*Proprietary formula/brand name

Depression

If you're feeling severely depressed, you should probably consult a mental health professional or psychopharmacologist. You might also want to consult a nutritionist. Most people suffer from varying degrees of depression during the course of a lifetime. Some of us bounce back more easily than others. If you are one of those who have difficulty bouncing back, there are solutions.

One thing I personally recommend is exercise. As a long-time runner and a three-time participant in the New York City

Marathon, I know firsthand that exercise has a powerful effect on mood and energy. Exercise increases the level of endorphins, which are chemicals in the brain that produce a "natural high." This high often lasts long after the exercise is over.

Also helpful in reducing depression is exposure to light on a regular basis. The lack of sunlight has a proven detrimental effect on mood. It appears that light, especially sunlight (and simulated sunlight), increases the level of serotonin, which has a calming effect on the psyche.

Here are some supplements I recommend as mood enhancers, along with recommended dosages:

Supplement	Amount per day
St. John's Wort	600 mg
NADH	2.5–5 mg
SAM	400 mg

Yeast

Do you suffer from any of these symptoms: fatigue, bloating, headaches, PMS, gas, bad breath, fungal infections, vaginal infections, recurrent bladder infections, itching, acne, eczema, psoriasis? Any one of these ailments could be a symptom of an overgrowth of yeast in your system. Your digestive system, particularly your colon, contains intestinal flora, including two types of bacteria: the "flowers," or *Lactobacillus acidophilus*, and the "weeds," or coliform bacteria.

Weeds are always going to grow in your garden, but you want to keep them under control. When the weeds become overgrown, they kill off the flowers. Yeast thrives in this garden of overgrown weeds. In fact, there are hundreds of types of yeast and fungi that grow inside us all the time. The most common and most prolific type of yeast is *Candida albicans*, which is generally found in the gastrointestinal tract and the genital area. When yeast thrives, it changes into a fungus with "roots" that bore tiny holes into the walls of the gastrointestinal tract. That allows the fungus—and the toxin it produces—to escape into the bloodstream.

The factors that promote the growth of yeast are the overconsumption of sugar, other carbohydrates, and yeast-containing products; treatment with antibiotics for an extended period of time; and use of oral contraceptives.

Because the symptoms of an overgrowth of yeast (also known as candida) are reminiscent of many other ailments, most people don't even know they have this condition. If you have any of the symptoms mentioned, try eliminating the foods that might be a contributing factor. If you're following the Balance plan, you have already begun to eliminate many of the agents that can cause yeast problems. There are also supplements you can take to "kill off" some of the weeds in your intestinal garden:

Supplement	Amount per day
Acidophilus	1/2 teaspoon
Olive leaf extract	100 mg
Grapefruit seed oil capsules	1000 mg

MENTAL FUNCTION

People seem to believe that as we grow older we must lose some of our mental abilities. It is true that age does some damage. We know about the harm that free radicals can do to all our cells, including brain cells. We are also exposed to so many pollutants and toxins over our lifetime that we can't help but suffer some of the consequences. If we continue to eat foods that produce harmful toxins, if we drink too much alcohol or smoke too many cigarettes, we do even more damage.

But—and this is a big but—many scientists now believe that it is not the actual aging process that results in loss of mental acuity; rather, the cause seems to be a decrease in mental activity. If you want to keep your brain in good shape, you have to exercise it. "Right up to the end of life, the more you challenge your brain, the more you can increase [the number of connections]," says neuroscientist Dr. Arnold Scheibel of the University of California, Los Angeles. "With a good deal of intellectual challenge you may be able to hold your own." In other words, "use it or lose it."

In addition to keeping up your mental activity, there are some supplements you can take to enhance your mental performance:

Supplement	Amount per day
Acetyl-L-carnitine	1000 mg
Ginkgo biloba	500 mg
Choline	100 mg
St. John's Wort	600 mg
Pregnenolone	20 mg
DMAE	250 mg

Cardiovascular Health

My basic recommendation for maintaining a healthy heart is to follow the Balance diet and exercise program. Your heart is a muscle that needs blood and oxygen to survive. If any of the passageways that provide either of these elements are blocked, damage—and sometimes death—will follow. Taking supplements can help keep your heart healthy, but they cannot substitute for the basic care you must provide through your daily intake of food and through exercising regularly. That said, following are some supplements that may be beneficial to your cardiovascular health:

Supplement	Amount per day
Omega-3 oils or flaxseed oil	1000 mg
Folic acid	200 micrograms
Vitamin B5	100 mg
Vitamin B6	100 mg
Vitamin B12	250 micrograms
DMG	125 mg
Coenzyme Q-10	30–60 mg
Garlic	500 mg
Magnesium	100 mg
Pantethine	250 mg
Vitamin E acetate	400 IU

LIFE EXTENSION

The final list of supplements is for what I call general life extension. These can be used to counteract the effects of living a long (and even healthy) life: too much exposure to the sun, the long-term effects of stress on your body, the natural loss of muscle mass that comes with aging, damage to the skin. These supplements can help you slow down the aging process:

Supplement	Amount per day
Vitamin E	400 IU
Alpha lipoic acid	100 mg
Vitamin C	1000 mg
Grape seed extract	100 mg
Bilberry	30 mg
Lutein	300 mg
Green tea extract	300 mg
Ginkgo biloba	500 mg
Saw palmetto (for men)	500 mg

The Balance

This chapter may seem a bit overwhelming. There are so many supplements available, so many new discoveries every day. And I have been talking only about cutting edge supplements in this chapter; I didn't even touch on most of the old standbys like calcium, rosehips, and zinc. You can't take everything or you'd be spending your entire day swallowing pills and powders. I offer this information to help you deal with specific problems you may be having; once those problems are solved, you can stop taking the corresponding supplements and start taking others that have more general health benefits.

12

THE BODY AND MIND IN BALANCE

For me, the journey toward The Balance has been an amazing adventure. It has involved two decades of observation, beginning with the origins of the modern holistic health movement and the rise of the human potential movement in the 1960s and 1970s.

Everywhere I looked, I saw people out of balance. I saw the imbalance of the culture at large, in the ways people dealt with stress and in the manner in which they lived their lives. I saw the imbalances within myself and within my family. I was desperate to find a better way to live my life. My journey started with the terrible migraine headaches I experienced on a regular basis, a legacy passed down from my mother. The only solution I was given from the medical establishment was to rely on a little pill that wasn't a cure at all, but a means of dealing with the pain.

I already knew from watching my mother that these drugs couldn't solve the underlying problem. She became addicted to pain killers, and twenty years later she was still suffering from migraines. I wanted to alleviate her suffering, and I did not want to suffer myself. Seeking answers, I found only a poverty of information. The doctors could tell me only to take the pain killers and to seek psychological help. But following this advice didn't stop the headaches from coming, and it didn't stop the fear that at any moment another one could begin.

My investigations led me to the field in which I have been working for the past twenty years. The understanding that traditional medicine has limitations opened up a whole new universe for me, an entire vocabulary of well-being. I changed my diet. I began to exercise. I gave up the overconsumption of stimulants such as coffee and alcohol. I began to move myself out of the up-and-down cycle of living the "crazy" life and to set myself up for the serenity of the balance of mind and body.

I think that mind and body in balance represents the transformational moment we're all looking for. We want something more than just a diet, more than another exercise program. Perhaps what we're looking for is a way to maintain a healthy lifestyle in the real world, a world in which stress comes with the territory, in which chemical pollutants are everywhere, in which the temptations of fat, sugar, and other processed carbohydrates are everywhere we turn.

To achieve a healthy lifestyle, you're going to have to pay greater attention to the subtleties of your personal care. It means you can't go through your life as carelessly as you have been. You have to be better prepared—psychologically, biologically, and metabolically. The demands on each of us are higher than they've ever been, and we must be prepared to fight for our lives.

Keeping your body in balance requires mixing and matching aspects of the Balance program, trying various combinations of diet, exercise, and supplements until you find the perfect fit for you. It means keeping your eye on the big picture all the time, whether you're at work or at play. How do you start your day? Do you wake up tired and need a powerful caffeine stimulant? Do you immediately throw your body into a state of alarm by drinking coffee? Do you give your body the fuel it needs, or do you skip breakfast and grab a Danish on your way to work? For me, the best way to get myself going is to start the day with exercise. Even if it's fifteen minutes or a half hour running in the park or on a treadmill at the gym or in your home, you can begin your day oxygenated and loaded with endorphins that will help you feel good for hours.

How do you deal with your day at work? Do you respond to stress by reaching for a chocolate bar? Or do you plan your meals for the workday, with healthy snacks between breakfast and lunch, and between lunch and dinner? If you want to keep yourself in balance and maintain optimum performance levels, you must plan your week in advance, preparing foods to take with you if necessary. You must take note of what healthy, metabolically correct foods are available to you in your office canteen or the neighborhood sandwich shop or restaurant.

Have you designed a program of supplements to deal with specific problems and to help maintain your general health? Part of the Balance program is protecting your neurological and nutritional health by taking advantage of all the latest breakthroughs in "neutraceuticals," which is the use of nutritional supplements for healing purposes. In examining these factors in my own life, I transformed my perspective concerning how I live my life, which engendered a transformation in my personal care. I'm hoping The Balance will do the same for you.

All the information in this book is meant to help you become a stronger, more capable human being. It is meant to show you ways to manage your weight by eating appropriately for your metabolic type, so that you are focusing on your overall health and personal care and not on losing weight. The focus is on living your life with health and vitality, getting the best possible performance from your mind and body.

Roger W. came into my office two years ago wearing dark glasses in a well-lit room. He was obviously on edge; his leg was shaking rapidly as he sat there. Stress was etched into the lines on his face. I asked him how it was he had come to see me. He told me several people had recommended this visit after noticing how stressed out he had become. Several years earlier, he said, he had inherited a successful business from his father and that had only increased his stress level. His weight was getting out of control.

I asked him what he had for breakfast that morning. He told me three or four fried eggs, some pork sausage, brown toast, and two cups of black coffee. He had two more cups of coffee midmorning. For lunch he had a turkey sandwich and two more cups of black coffee. Just before he came to my office, he had a chocolate bar. He added that he would probably have another two cups of coffee before he went to see his therapist later that night.

I asked him if he was happy. "I don't know what that means," he replied. "I'm usually in a bad mood. I'm chronically depressed." He told me he saw his therapist two or three times a week. His life, he said, consisted of going to work, going to therapy, and going home.

After his recent divorce, he had moved into a new flat. I asked him to describe it. "I've got a mattress on top of a box spring," he said. "And there are boxes everywhere because I haven't unpacked yet."

We worked together for two years. The first and most dramatic step was to wean Roger off coffee. He had a difficult time, and for a while his depression deepened. But then I got him to join a health club and to get a massage once a week to relieve some of his stress. He decreased his therapy sessions to once a week. There is nothing inherently wrong with therapy, but much of his depression was related to the biochemical imbalances he was experiencing.

Roger dropped nearly three stone. Just recently I ran into him eating dinner in a health food restaurant. He introduced me to his fiancée. He was not wearing dark glasses. He told me that he had finally unpacked his boxes. He was a different human being. "And," he said, "I am finally happy."

Roger's story represents the ultimate goals in life. It is not about how much money you have or how much you weigh. It is about how much of yourself you can "unpack" and share with others. It is getting out from behind those dark glasses, looking life right in the eye, and having the strength and energy to enjoy it. It is striving for your peak performance level at a pace that is comfortable for you. It is how good you feel, in your body and in your mind.

APPENDIX

Appendix A

GLOSSARY OF SUPPLEMENTS

The following list of supplements and products is by no means a complete one, nor is the information on each supplement meant to be encyclopedic. In our lectures and seminars and in our private consulting practice, both my partner Jonathan Bowden, M.A., and I consistently stand as patient advocates and for patient responsibility. We want the people we work with to collaborate on their health care with their health care practitioners.

Our purpose is to inform and educate people about their options and opportunities. In that spirit we present the following information, in the hopes that it will alert you to some of the interesting compounds that are available and may be of use to you in your own journey toward vibrant well-being, optimal health, and a body and a life in Balance.

Acetyl-L-Carnitine (see also carnitine): This is a kind of "super-carnitine" that is both better absorbed and more active than the "plain" kind. It is used to improve mood and mental energy, and as an anti-aging compound for brain cells. There is solid research on using acetyl-L-carnitine with the elderly, both for depression and for the slowing of Alzheimer's, and it appears to have no negative side effects. It is, however, expensive. Generally healthy people can use it in combination with carnitine to improve mental and physical performance. Caution should be taken by epileptics, since they are already sensitive to neural stimulation.

Acidophilus: A normal, healthy colon contains a balance of two types of bacteria: the "good guy" is *Lactobacillus acidophilus*, and the "bad guy" is coliform bacteria. An imbalance in these bacteria can occur from over-consumption of carbohydrates and sugar, from yeast, from taking antibiotics for an extended period of time, or from taking oral contraceptives. Taking a supplement of *Lactobacillus acipdophilus* can help restore the proper balance in your system.

Alpha Lipoic Acid: This recently discovered substance, also known as lipoic acid and thioctic acid, is a powerful antioxidant which is effective against a wider range of free radicals than either vitamin E or vitamin C. It either protects or mimics the actions of other antioxidants. It is easy to absorb and assimilate. It may help to improve energy metabolism, particularly in people with diabetes, liver cirrhosis or heart disease. Alpha lipoic acid aids in the conversion of food into energy, and has been used in Germany as an approved drug for the treatment of diabetic neuropathy. Alpha lipoic acid also is thought to be a powerful protector of the liver; a recent study showed that when rats were given a known carcinogen, those that were also given alpha lipoic acid developed significantly less liver cancer than those that were not.

Bilberry: A cousin of the blueberry, the bilberry contains anthocyanosides which are potent antioxidants important for the health of the eyes.

Branched Chain Amino Acids: Branched Chain Amino Acids are three specific acids: Leucine, Isoleucine, and Valine, which are often considered "muscle fuel" because they are found in high amounts in the muscle cells, and tend to be used as fuel during high intensity exercise. Stress—including high intensity exercise—appears to deplete these amino acids, and many athletes supplement them with a BCAA formula.

Carnitine: Carnitine, or L-Carnitine, is an amino acid made in the body from the essential amino acids lysine and methionine. In foods, it is found mostly in meat, especially in beef. Its job is to "escort" fatty acids from the bloodstream into the mitochondria, where they get burned for energy. It has frequently been associated with weight loss. The theory is that extra carnitine can help this fat burning process work more efficiently, though the exact way this works is still unknown. In any case, carnitine does help your cells produce energy. It is found in the heart more than in any other part of the body. Extra carnitine may be helpful for people with angina or heart conditions, and it may also help with chronic fatigue, with improving cholesterol levels and lowering blood triglycerides. Incidentally, it's indispensable for infants, who usually get it from breast milk. If you use formula, make sure the formula is fortified with carnitine.

Carotinoids: This family of compounds includes the carotenes (found in many orange and red colored fruits and vegetables) and xanthophylls (found in dark-green leafy vegetables). They are powerful antioxidants; some, like beta-carotene and lycopene, appear to have a protective effect against cancer; others, like lutein, also protect your eyes against free radical damage. Beta-carotene, the most famous of the carotenes, "turns on" immune cells, and fights cancer and infection.

Choline: Choline is a coenzyme (it helps enzymes do their work) that aids in metabolism. Researchers think that choline may help to preserve the brain's ability to reason, learn, and remember. It has also been shown to improve the memory in Alzheimer's patients.

Coenzyme Q-10: Dr. Robert Atkins says that when he coined the term "vita-nutrient" he was thinking of Coenzyme Q-10. This nutrient is absolutely vital to good health, is essential to energy production and to longer cell life. It is one of the most powerful antioxidants, and has been shown to be extremely effective in several studies investigating its effects on heart failure patients. The high energy needs of the heart make this organ a natural beneficiary of CoQ-10's health giving properties and it contains twice as much of this nutrient as any other organ or tissue in the body. CoQ-10 has also been used for treating high blood pressure, high blood sugar, and is believed to have a rejuvenating effect on the immune system.

Conjugated Linoleic Acid: CLA has been researched primarily for its powerful anti-carcinogenic properties. In addition it has dramatic effects in regulating and reducing body fat in animals. Other studies using supplemental CLA in the diets of animals have shown significant drops in blood concentrations of total cholesterol and "bad" LDL, and a reduction in chemically induced cancers. CLA is one of the few animal derived "natural substances" that has been shown to have anti-cancer benefits.

Animal research has recently shown that CLA has a potent ability to regulate body fat accumulation and retention. Though human studies do not yet exist, animal studies are very promising; laboratory animals consuming controlled amounts of CLA have shown significant decreases in body fat, as well as increases in lean body mass.

CLA is actually an isomer, a chemically altered form of one of the essential fatty acids, linoleic acid. But humans cannot convert linoleic acid to conjugated linoleic acid; they must rely instead on getting it from the diet (or from supplements). It's found in animal-derived foods—the highest amounts are in meats and dairy products. Since the CLA content of foods has dropped nearly 80 percent in the past 20 years, largely due to changes in livestock feeding methods, CLA may turn out to be a terrific addition to the supplement arsenal for both its fat regulating properties and for its positive effects on cancer and cholesterol levels.

Chromium: This important mineral has a critical function in the body: it helps insulin to do its job more effectively. What this means is that the body may require less insulin to do the same job, i.e., metabolizing sugar (glucose). This has profound implications for the management of blood sugar, cravings, and ultimately, fat storage. Researchers have found that diabetics who take chromium can, in many cases, stabilize their blood sugar levels and reduce the amount of medication they need. Chromium is virtually absent from the soil, and difficult to absorb in any case (only about 3 percent of dietary chromium is retained in the body). Systematic deficiency is common in the United States.

Creatine Monohydrate: Creatine Monohydrate is probably the most popular supplement in body building and enjoys an exalted reputation among athletes in general for its ability to increase strength. Creatine is a compound that is made in our bodies and converted to an energy compound in the muscles known as creatine phosphate. It can be found in food; red meat is the best source. The short explanation is that the more creatine in the muscle, the longer you can perform a high intensity exercise—like a set of squats or bench presses or a sprint—before reaching muscle exhaustion. The theory goes that by loading up on creatine (thus increasing stores in the body), we can perform an exercise with greater intensity before reaching failure, thus allowing for significant gains in strength. Creatine continues to be investigated by researchers in exercise physiology and sports performance, and the overall verdict remains quite positive.

Dandelion: The leaves, roots, and tops of the dandelion plant are used in herbal medicine for a variety of purposes. Dandelion acts as a general detoxifier, cleansing the bloodstream and liver. It is also a mild diuretic and can help reduce fluid retention. The root is better as a detoxifier; the extract of the leaves better for fluid retention.

DHA: Docosahexaenoic acid (DHA) is an omega-3 fatty acid. Omegas are a special class of polyunsaturated fats, some of which, like DHA, are considered very valuable for human health. The body makes DHA from the essential fatty acid, linolenic acid, but the main dietary sources are fish and fish oils.

DHEA: This is a hormone produced by the adrenal glands. Levels of DHEA decrease in the body beginning around the age of twenty. This decrease appears to be a factor in many age-related diseases and disorders. Studies suggest that people with high DHEA levels live longer and have less heart disease and cancer. DHEA is useful in many areas related to memory loss, recall, and for improving long-term memory. It increases estrogen production in women and testosterone in men to levels found in younger people. Because DHEA is a precursor of testosterone and estrogen and can cause elevated levels of these hormones, it should be taken only after consulting a health professional.

DMAE: Dimethylaminoethanol (DMAE), is a precursor to choline, and has also been called a "smart drug." It enhances brain and memory function. According to some writers in the field, DMAE has shown promise as an effective treatment for children with Attention Deficit Disorder (ADD) and may be a natural alternative to the much-prescribed Ritalin.

DMG (dimethylglycene): Dimethylglycine is a metabolic enhancer. Technically, this interesting nutrient is a "methyl donor," which means it combines in the body with a single extra carbon cluster, converting into a chemical that, according to Dr. Robert Atkins "neutralizes toxins and protects our genes." DMG appears to be a valuable "pick-me-up" useful for run of the mill fatigue and increasing energy and stamina. It is also a detoxifying agent and shows promise as an antioxidant and booster of immune system function. Runners frequently use sublingual DMG while doing long distance events; preliminary observations indicate that athletes can exercise longer before becoming physically exhausted when supplementing with only 5 mg of this nutrient.

Dong Quai: An herb that has been used in the treatment of female problems like the menopause, PMS, and hot flashes. Like evening primrose oil, it can have a balancing effect on ovarian hormones.

Echinacea: This herb comes from a North American wildflower used more than any other by Native Americans for its reported immune enhancing actions. It is especially helpful in fighting off winter colds. It has also been used to help heal wounds; echinaecea is a substance that knits skin and prevents germs from penetrating tissues). It is an effective antiobiotic and anti-inflammatory agent.

Folic Acid (also B6 and B12): After 25 years of research, Dr. Kilmer McCully of Harvard University finally achieved mainstream recognition when the powers that be recognized his pioneering work in the area of homocysteine. It is an artery-wall damaging amino acid that can build up in the bloodstream. High levels of homocysteine tend to run in families. Homocysteine is now recognized as a risk factor for heart disease independent of cholesterol or any other risk factors. In fact, many researchers and theorists believe that it will eventually eclipse cholesterol as the number one risk factor for heart disease and almost every form of arteriosclerosis.

Folic acid, one of the B vitamins, is probably one of the most efficient methods of reducing homocysteine levels. We believe that as research continues, more and more degenerative and other disorders will be found to have a connection to elevated homocysteine levels.

Folic acid is vital to the development of the nervous system in the fetus and has long been recognized as a preventative for neural tube birth defects (spina bifida) and even mainstream medicine now recommends that every woman of childbearing age maintain adequate folic acid intake. Taking folic acid, along with vitamins B6 and B12, is probably one of the most efficient methods of reducing homocysteine levels.

Garlic: This is one of the most potent antioxidant foods (and supplements) which may be helpful as a weapon against high cholesterol and arteriosclerosis. A sulfur compound found in aged garlic may have a protective effect against cancer; other garlic compounds seem to have the effect of lowering blood pressure.

Ginkgo Biloba: This herb has demonstrated remarkable effects in improving many symptoms associated with aging. It can help delay and in some cases reverse the mental deterioration in the early stages of Alzheimer's. It increases circulation in the brain, and can improve memory loss, brain function, and depression.

Glutathione: Glutathione is one of the stars on the antioxidant playing field. It's an amino acid, and is considered by many to be one of the most powerful anti-aging nutrients ever discovered. Apparently, glutathione "picks up" any toxic substances that have found their way into your body and escorts them out. It is a tripeptide, that is, a small protein made from three amino acids: cysteine, glycine, and glutamic acid. You also need sulfur (contained in the cysteine) and selenium to make it. Fish oil may also help your body produce more glutathione.

As we age, most of us have declining glutathione levels. There is some controversy about the best way to raise glutathione levels in the body, though there is little controversy that raising the levels is a desirable thing. (This is because some of the glutathione you take in a supplement gets broken down into its amino acids by your digestive juices.) You can supplement with glutathione directly, or by taking cysteine (see N-Acetyl-Cysteine), or by taking glutamine (which stimulates your liver to make more glutathione).

Glutathione has been investigated as a potential suppressant of the HIV virus, at least in the test tube, by researchers in Harvard, Stanford, and elsewhere. Many complementary medicine centers use it as an important part of treatment for patients with Chron's and ulcerative colitis. Glutathione plays a critical role in defending the body against free radical damage, helps prevent cataracts and other eye conditions, and perhaps most important, is a significant booster of the immune system.

Goldenseal Root: Goldenseal was one of the favorite herbs of the Cherokees of North America. It has a positive effect on the mucous membranes and body tissues. It is excellent for problems of the nose, throat, and bronchial passages, and is helpful in clearing nasal congestion. There are, however, warnings against goldenseal for pregnant women and for people who suffer from high blood pressure or heart disease.

Gotu Kola: This herb is a well-known remedy used in Ayurvedic (Eastern Indian) medicine. It has just recently become widely available in the United States. It heals the underlying structure of the skin's tissue and promotes new skin growth. It is very good for treating skin and connective tissue damage. The active substances in gotu kola are believed to be steroid-like compounds called tripertenes, which seem to have a balancing effect on connective tissue. It also contains a group of triterpenes called asiaticosides which possess strong antioxidant properties and stimulate healthy skin. Gotu kola stimulates hair and nail growth, increases blood supply to connective tissue, enhances connective tissue structure, and reduces scar tissue.

Grapefruit Seed Oil: This is a botanical extract made from the seeds and pulp of grapefruits. It has been found to be helpful in aiding with digestion and helping ease colds, flus, and sore throats. It is also sometimes recommended for relief of symptoms associated with yeast problems. It is usually taken in liquid form, mixed with juice or herbal teas. Since this extract is fairly new on the supplement scene, check with your physician or nutritionist before trying it to get the proper dosage.

Green Tea Extract: This herbal extract contains polyphenols, potent antioxidants which have been shown to significantly lower the risks of many diseases including cancer, heart disease, and stroke. Green tea extract protects against and may be an effective treatment for many common degenerative diseases.

HMB: HMB (an abbreviation for "beta hydroxy beta-methylbutyrate") is one of the more interesting supplements to come along in a long time. Many studies support its ability to help you gain lean muscle mass and increase strength in conjunction with a good resistance training program. It has been found to have a consistent, positive effect on protein metabolism, and appears to be non-toxic and very safe. It is not entirely clear at this time exactly how HMB supports muscle building. One hypothesis is that it may supply certain compounds to the muscle and to the immune system that result in maximal repair after exercise. It is also hypothesized that HMB works as a kind of "anti-catabolic," i.e., it helps support a decrease in muscle damage or muscle breakdown. Regardless, this supplement seems to produce very promising results for those on a muscle and strength building program.

Huperzine A: This compound, derived from club moss tea, has been reputed to have potent abilities to enhance memory. Studies carried out in China indicate that it shows promise as a part of treatment for Alzheimer's and senile memory deficits.

Inositol and Inositol Hexaphosphate: Inositol is closely associated with choline. In combination with choline, it helps the liver to process fat. It is also found to be useful in brain cell nutrition. The spinal cord nerves, the brain, and the cerebral fluid all contain large quantities of inositol, and it is needed for the growth and survival of cells in many places in the body. Inositol levels are often lower in people hospitalized for depression. Recently, a form of inositol called inositol hexaphosphate has been investigated for its remarkable anti-tumor effects and general positive effect on the immune system.

Light Therapy: Light therapy has been used for the treatment of "winter depression" for about a decade. Very respected researchers have found that many depressive symptoms can literally lighten up within days of treatment. The real buzz is that it appears that exposure to light may stimulate serotonin. This is an easy, non-invasive treatment many people have found helpful.

Lutein: A form of carotenoid found in dark-green leafy vegetables which helps protect your eyes against free radical damage.

Lycopene: A member of the carotenoid family that includes beta-carotene, lycopene may be one of the most potent antioxidants of all. It is specifically known for its ability to trap cancer-promoting free radicals. Some of the best sources of lycopene are tomatoes, tomato sauces, grapefruit, and watermelon.

L-tyrosine: This amino acid has been shown to aid in the treatment of anxiety, depression, and allergies. It acts as a mood elevator and stress reliever.

Magnesium: Magnesium is involved in many essential metabolic processes, including the production of glucose and protein. It is also involved in muscle impulse transmission and neurotransmission and activity. Magnesium helps promote absorption and metabolism of other minerals such as calcium, phosphorus, sodium, and potassium. It aids during bone growth and is necessary for proper functioning of the muscles, including the heart. Magnesium is vital in helping to prevent heart attacks. Research has shown that patients who take magnesium after a heart attack have a much better survival rate. Magnesium has also been found effective for treating PMS. Many people in the American alternative health field estimate that anywhere from 70–80 percent of people take in less than the optimal level of magnesium. Some integrative medicine pioneers point out that magnesium is nature's own "calcium channel blocker."

MCT (MCT oil): MCT stands for "medium-chain triglycerides," a form of fat which is different from LCTs ("long-chain triglycerides") which are the most abundant fats found in nature. LCTs are the storage fat for humans. MCTs on the other hand, can be rapidly burned by the body as energy and can actually promote accessing and burning of fat stores in the body.

MCTs are thought to increase the rate at which calories burn (thermogenesis). The purpose is to take in enough calories to maintain body weight and energy, thus preventing the body from breaking down protein (muscle) for energy. Taking MCTs accomplishes this without the "side effects" of extra carbohydrate (water retention, insulin spikes, etc.). Although technically a fat, the body seems to prefer using MCT as if it were a carbohydrate and burns it preferentially as fuel. Dieters take MCTs for the same reasons, namely that they appear to have a thermogenic effect.

Melatonin: Melatonin is the active hormone secreted by the pineal gland, a small gland found inside your brain. The pineal gland controls what's called the "circadian rhythms" — your body's sleep-wake cycles and internal sense of time. Melatonin has been touted as a world class antioxidant, protecting us from two of the worst free radicals, peroxyl and hydroxyl. More conservative researchers feel the claims being made for melatonin's anti-aging properties, its possible shield against cancer, heart disease, and neurological conditions, remain to be seen. But nearly everyone agrees that it is enormously helpful in the area of sleep. Our bodies begin to make melatonin at the beginning of darkness. After the age of 40, you make less and less of it. If you can't drift off to sleep when at rest, melatonin is one of the best and safest solutions.

Milk Thistle: Milk thistle contains the active flavonoid silymarin. It is effective against all liver disorders, and contains some of the most potent liver protecting substances ever discovered. It stimulates the production of new liver cells and prevents formation of a damaging class of eicosanoids called leukotrienes. Daily supplementation of 150–300 mg encourages the liver to make glutathione, one of the body's best natural antioxidants, and higher dosages are used to treat liver disease. Cenegenics, one of the top anti-aging clinics in the United States, routinely uses milk thistle in its daily supplement preparations as an overall detoxifier and liver protector.

NAC (N-Acetylcysteine): NAC is a precursor of L-Glutathione in the body. It is a sulfur-containing amino acid, and is a very potent antioxidant and detoxifier.

NADH: Reduced B-nicotinamide adenine dinucleotide (NADH) is a co-enzyme, which means it is a substance which makes it possible for certain enzymes to do their work in the body. NADH is a "cutting edge" supplement that is currently being researched for its positive effects on Alzheimer's, Parkinson's, and Chronic Fatigue Syndrome. It is best known as a substance that improves athletic endurance, and is thought to energize body and brain activity, improve alertness, concentration, emotions, drive, and overall mood.

Olive Leaf Extract: Olive leaf kills germs and is a preventative against colds, flu, the mumps, and many other infections; it is also antifungal, antiparasitic, and antimicrobial.

Omega-3s and -6s/ Essential Fatty Acids: The list of health conditions that can benefit from essential fatty acid supplementation is too long to list. Essential fatty acid deficiencies are implicated in a wide variety of conditions. Imbalances between the two, pandemic in the Western diet, may have a causative role in arthritis and other degenerative diseases. The absence of essential fatty acids may contribute to difficulty in losing weight. One omega-6, GLA, has been found to help in the treatment of PMS; another omega-3, DHA (found in fish oils) can be used directly by the brain. Diets high in omega-3 fatty acids can prevent heart attacks, lower blood pressure, and lower cholesterol and triglyceride levels. (Review chapter 7 for more information about essential fatty acids.)

Pantethine (Vitamin B5): Pantothenic acid is part of the vitamin B complex; pantethine is a metabolite of panthothenic acid. Pantethine research shows that it is a cholesterol-lowering agent that will aid in cardiovascular disease.

Phosphatidylserine: Look for a lot of information to be coming out on this very promising phospholipid. Phospholipids hold cells together and also control the movement of substances into the cells. Phosphatidylserine is an extremely important phospholipid that is intimately involved in relaying chemical messages throughout the brain (where it is found in large amounts). It also helps brain cells to retrieve information and to store information; and it declines significantly as we age. Its supporters claim superb results in improvement of brain function and memory.

Pregnenelone: Pregnenelone is the hormone from which DHEA and almost all sex steroid hormones are made in the body. It is therefore a precursor to testosterone, estrogen, cortisol and aldosterone. It is particularly useful to women because it can lead to the production of progesterone, creating a balance with estrogen which can reduce the risk of certain cancers.

Pyruvate: Preliminary studies have shown that pyruvate increases muscular endurance by enhancing the transport of glucose into the muscle cells. It has also been shown to increase fat utilization. Right now, the only drawback to using pyruvate for fat loss is the extremely large amounts that seem to be necessary to get the job done. Personal correspondence with some of the leading researchers in the field, however, indicate that several companies are currently working on a form of pyruvate that may be effective at much smaller dosages. Additional research is ongoing, and we may be hearing more about this supplement in the future.

SAM (s-adenosylmethionine): SAM has been used in Europe as an anti-depressant drug for many years. It has almost no side effects. Its proponents believe it to be one of the safest, most effective antidepressants in the world. It is also thought to offer significant support for liver function. It has been found to protect against osteoarthritis, and also to reduce levels of homocysteine, and may be useful in preventing heart disease. You should not take SAM if you are already taking prescription anti-depressant drugs.

Saw Palmetto Extract (and Pygeum): This is one of the most effective agents in treating benign prostate hyperplasia, a major medical problem for older men. Over twenty studies conducted according to the most rigorous, double-blind standards of conservative journal publication have shown that saw palmetto is superior to the prescription drug Proscar for treating benign prostrate enlargement. I recommend that every man over 40 take saw palmetto extract. Pygeum, which comes from the bark of a tropical tree, is also effective for the prostate, relieving urinary problems and other symptoms. Many formulas contain both extracts.

Selenium: An essential mineral, selenium is a natural antioxidant that protects against free radicals. It is thought to contribute to the prevention of many diseases, including cancer, arteriosclerosis, stroke, cirrhosis, arthritis and emphysema. It is even more effective in combination with vitamin E.

Soy Isoflavinoids: Soy products contain isoflavones, hormone-like substances which have been found to help prevent breast cancer. Soybean foods such as soy milk, tofu, and miso could well be the cheapest and easiest protection against breast and prostate cancer; they also contain phytoestrogens, hormone-like compounds found in plants, which have been shown to modulate the unpleasant effects of menopause. In addition, soy products help keep cholesterol down.

St. John's Wort: This herb has been used to effectively combat mild to moderate forms of depression — without the side effects (such as sexual dysfunction) of prescription drugs. It contains the active ingredient hypericin, and has long been used in Germany as an anti-depressant. It's recommended that it not be taken with other anti-depressants without a health professional's go-ahead, and there is no evidence that it will help with severe depression or manic-depressive illness. However, it does keep serotonin levels elevated.

Recently it has begun to be used in conjunction with phentermine and essential amino acids at the Institute for Medical Weight Loss in Tucson, Arizona. This combination seems to decrease the craving for carbohydrates and salt-based foods, but it is not completely clear how the mechanism works. If you take St. John's Wort, you should be cautious about exposing yourself to sunlight, especially if you're fair skinned. The herb also has high concentrations of immune-stimulating chemicals known as flavonoids.

Trimethylglycine: Trimethylglycine (TMG) donates its three methyl groups to accomplish the conversion of homocysteine into methionine and SAM. TMG is said to lower homocysteine levels. Research is now showing that lowering homocysteine levels protects against a wide variety of ills associated with aging, including heart disease, cancer, and liver diseases.

Vitamin C: This is one of the most potent antioxidants; dozens of studies have documented its protective effect against cancers, heart disease, cataracts, and many other serious health problems. It helps bolster the immune system and it also enhances the effectiveness of other antioxidants such as vitamin E.

Vitamin E: Although vitamin E is potent antioxidant, it is difficult to get from foods in large enough amounts to have a therapeutic effect. It has been shown to decrease the risk of heart attacks, slow the progression of Alzheimer's disease, and increase immunity in the elderly. Supplemental vitamin E protects brain and nerve cells against free radical damage. Animal studies indicate that it may also have a protective effect against breast cancer.

Whey Peptide: Whey peptide (or whey protein) powders are one of the best additions to the supplement arsenal for a number of reasons. They answer the question often asked by clients, "How do I get more protein into my diet?" and they do it in a way that is convenient, easy, and inexpensive. Whey protein is one of the easiest to assimilate, highest quality proteins available; it's biological value (BV) is among the highest of any protein. It has a very high concentration of essential amino acids. In addition, many high-end whey protein powders are fortified with glutamine, an amino acid of great importance to muscle building and preservation. Whey is the run-off of the cheese making process; high quality whey proteins have the lactose removed, resulting in a product that is easily tolerated, easily mixed into shakes, has virtually no fat, and is pretty tasty as well. Add to that the fact that it now appears that whey protein has additional benefits: it boosts glutathione levels and appears improve immune response.

Appendix B

RESOURCE GUIDE

Please note that the following listing is for information only and does not imply any endorsement, nor do the organizations listed necessarily agree with the views expressed in this book.

AUSTRALIA AND NEW ZEALAND

Australian Natural Therapists Association
Tel: 1800 817 577
www.Anta.com.au

Australian Traditional Medicine Society
PO Box 1027
Meadowbank
NSW 114
Tel: 02 9809 6800
www.atms.com.au

The New Zealand Charter of Health Practitioners Inc.
PO Box 36–588
Northcote
Auckland
Tel: 09 443 6255
Fax: 09 443 2336
www.healthcharter.org.nz

UK

British Council of Complementary Medicine
PO Box 2074
Seaford BN25 1HG
Tel: 0845 345 5977
Fax: 0845 345 5978
www.bcma.co.uk

British Nutrition Foundation
High Holborn House
52–54 High Holborn
London WC1V 6RQ
Tel: 020 7404 6504
Fax: 020 7404 6747
www.nutrition.org.uk

Health Development Authority
Tevelyan House
30 Great Peter Street
London SW1P 2HW
www.hda-online.org.uk

Institute for Optimum Nutrition
Blades Court
Deodar Road
London SW15 2NV
Tel: 020 8877 9993
Fax: 020 8877 9980
www.ion.ac.uk

Institute of Complementary Medicine
PO Box 194
London SE16 7QZ
Tel: 020 7237 5165
Fax: 020 7237 5175
www.icmedicine.co.uk

Society for the Promotion of Nutritional Therapy (SPNT)
www.waterfall2000.com/spnt

BIBLIOGRAPHY

"AGEs and Aging: A Definite Link That is Worth Breaking." *Life Extension Magazine.* Sept. 1997: 48.

Angier, Natalie. "Fat on Thighs and Paunches Is the Fate of All Mammals." *The New York Times.* Oct. 30, 1990: C1.

Arnot, Robert. *Dr. Arnot's Revolutionary Weight Control Program.* Boston: Little, Brown & Company, 1997.

Asterita, Mary F. *The Physiology of Stress.* Gary, IN: Human Sciences Press, Inc., 1985.

Atkins, Robert C. *Dr. Atkins' New Diet Revolution.* New York: M. Evans and Company, Inc., 1992.

———. *The Vita-Nutrient Solution.* New York: Simon and Schuster, 1998.

Bailey, Covert. *Smart Exercise: Burning Fat, Getting Fit.* Boston: Houghton Mifflin, 1994.

Balch, James F. and Phyllis A. Balch. *Prescription for Nutritional Healing.* Garden City Park, NY: Avery Publishing Group, Inc., 1990.

Begley, Sharon with Mary Hager. "The Search for the Fountain of Youth." *Newsweek.* March 5, 1990: 44–52.

"Benefit Found in Asian Diet with Fish Oil." *The New York Times.* Aug. 1, 1997: C5.

Bennet, William and Joel Gurin. "Do Diets Really Work?" *Science.* March, 1982: 42–50.

Brody, Jane. "Intriguing Studies Link Nutrition to Immunity." *The New York Times.* March 21, 1989: C1.

———. "Vitamin E Greatly Reduces Risk of Heart Disease, Studies Suggest." *The New York Times.* May 20, 1993: A1.

Charlier, Marj. "Cave Man's Life is Worth Aping, Doctors Believe." *The Wall Street Journal.* Oct. 21, 1986: 35.

"Coffee and Health." *Consumer Reports.* Oct. 1994: 650–52.

Colgan, Michael. *Optimum Sports Nutrition.* Ronkonkoma, NY: Advanced Research Press, 1993.

Cranton, Elmer M. and Arlene Brecher. *Bypassing Bypass.* Herndon, VA: Medex Publishing, Inc., 1984.

Cranton, Elmer M. and James P. Frackelton. "Free radical pathology in age-associated diseases." *Journal of Holistic Medicine.* Spring/Summer, 1984: 50–54.

Crowley, Geoffrey and Anne Underwood. "The Mood Controller: A Little Help from Serotonin." *Newsweek.* Dec. 29, 1997: 46–51.

D'Adamo, Peter H. with Catherine Whitney. *Eat Right 4 Your Type.* New York: G.P. Putnam's Sons, 1996.

Daniel, Jere. "Death-Defying Dieting: New Risks of Yo-Yoing." *Longevity*, April, 1989: 20–22.

Dufty, William. *Sugar Blues.* New York: Warner Books, 1975.

Eades, Michael R. and Mary Dean Eades. *Protein Power.* New York: Bantam Books, 1996.

Flippin, Royce. "How Exercise Works." *Self.* Jan. 1993: 77.

Fowkes, Steven Wm. "What are Free Radicals?" *Smart Drug News.* April 15, 1996: 2.

Fraser. Laura. *Losing It: America's Obsession with Weight and the Industry that Feeds on It.* New York: Dutton Books, 1997.

Garner, David M. "The 1997 Body Image Survey Results." *Psychology Today.* Jan/Feb. 1997: 30–36.

Gittleman, Ann Louise with James Templeton and Candelor Versace. *Your Body Knows Best*. New York: Pocket Books, 1997.

Gittleman, Ann Louise. *Super Nutrition for Women*. New York: Bantam Books, 1991.

Greenberg, Kurt. *Challenging Orthodoxy*. New Canaan, CT: Keats Publishing, 1991.

Grimes, William. "Self-Denial Takes a Holiday." *The New York Times*. Nov. 26, 1997: F1.

Grunwald, Lisa. "Do I Look Fat to You?" *Life*. Feb. 1995: 58–74.

Howell, Wanda H., McNamara, Donald J., Tosca, Mark A., Smith, Bruce T., and Gaines, John A. "Plasma lipid and lipoprotein responses to dietary fat and cholesterol: a meta-analysis." *American Journal of Clinical Nutrition*. June 1997; 65: 1464–74.

Kelley, William D. *The Metabolic Types*. Lake Geneva, WI: Computrition Investments, 1980.

Kirschman, Gayla J. and John D. Kirschman. *Nutrition Almanac*. New York: McGraw-Hill, 1996.

Krohn, Jacqueline, Taylor, Frances A., and Larson, Erla Mae. *The Whole Way to Allergy Relief and Prevention*. Point Roberts, WA: Hartley & Marks, 1991.

Lagua, Rosalina T. and Virginia S. Claudio, *Nutrition and Diet Therapy Reference Dictionary*. New York: Chapman and Hall, 1996.

Lemonick, Michael D. "The Mood Molecule." *Time Magazine*. Sept. 29, 1977: 74–82.

Lowey, Nita. "The Fight Against Eating Disorders." *Women's News*. Nov. 1997: 4.

Mayo, Joseph L. "Premenstrual Syndrome: A Natural Approach to Management." *Clinical Nutrition Insights*. July 1997: 1–7.

Mellin, Laurel. *The Solution: 6 Winning Ways to Permanent Weight Loss*. New York: ReganBooks, 1997.

Murray, Michael T. "A Comprehensive Evaluation of Premenstrual Syndrome." *American Journal of Natural Medicine*. March 1997: 6–19.

Murray, Michael, N.D. *Encyclopedia of Nutritional Supplements*. Ricklin, CA: Prima Publishing, 1996.

Nash, Madeline. "Addicted." *Time Magazine*. May 5, 1997: 69–76.

Null, Gary. *The Clinician's Handbook of Natural Healing*. New York: Kensington Books, 1997.

Pressman, Alan. *The Complete Idiot's Guide to Vitamins and Minerals*. New York: Simon and Schuster, 1997.

Pritikin, Nathan. *The Pritikin Promise: 28 Days to a Longer, Healthier Life*. New York: Pocket Books, 1982.

Quillin, Patrick. *Healing Nutrients*. New York: Vintage Books, 1989.

Rosenstock, Linda, Keifer, Matthew, Daniell, William E., et al. "Chronic central nervous system effects of acute organophosphate pesticide intoxication." *Lancet* 1991; 338: 223–27.

Schmidt, Karen F. "Old No More." *U.S. News and World Report*. March 8, 1993: 66–73.

Sears, Barry with Bill Lawren. *The Zone*. New York: ReganBooks, 1995.

Segell, Michael. "How to Live Forever." *Esquire*. Sept. 1993: 125–132.

Selye, Hans. *The Stress of Life*. New York: The McGraw-Hill Book Company, 1976.

Sheats, Cliff. *Lean Bodies*. New York: Warner Books, 1995.

Toufexis, Anastasia. "The New Scoop on Vitamins." *Time*. April 6, 1992: 54–59.

Waterhouse, Debra. *Outsmarting the Female Fat Cell*. Los Angeles: Time Warner AudioBooks, 1994.

Watts, David L. *Trace Elements and Other Essential Nutrients*. Dallas, TX: Trace Elements, Inc., 1995.

Williams, Roger J. *Biochemical Individuality*. Austin, TX: University of Texas Press, 1956.

INDEX

Abdominal fat, 80–81, 136
Addictive personalities, 136
Adrenal glands, 40, 41, 51, 62, 115, 134
Adrenaline, 41, 46, 134, 135
Aerobic exercise, 8, 84, 130–31, 148, 163
Aging:
  anti-aging supplements, 167, 176
  antioxidants and, 164–66
  reducing premature, 12, 71
  science of health and, 157–83
Alcohol, 16, 45, 48, 49, 84, 160
  eliminating or reducing excessive, 97
  stress and, 56
Allergies, 99
Allergy Research Group, 86
Alley, Kirstie, 76
All Natural Muscular Development, 170
Alternative medicine, xv
Alzheimer's disease, 70
American Journal of Clinical Nutrition, 110
Anabolism, 6
Angier, Natalie, 80
Animal protein:
  for fast burners, 140
  for slow burners, 121
Annual Review of Nutrition, 162
Anorexia nervosa, 74, 75
Antibiotics, 174
Antioxidants, 69–70, 164–66
  supplements, 165–66, 167
Anxiety, 55, 57–58, 65, 135
  free-floating, 48
Appetite, 9, 111, 124
  change in eating habits, 48
  satiety, 51–52
  stress and, 51–52
  see also Hunger
Apple-shaped body type, 80–81, 117, 136
Arteriosclerosis, 29, 37
Arthritis, 29, 47
Asterita, Mary, 134
Asthma, 47
Autism, 66
Ayurvedic medicine, 96

Back pain, 48
Bailey, Covert, 163
Balance, The:
  of body and mind, 179–83
  calorie counting and, 111
  defined, 6, 8
  effectiveness of, reason for, 13–15
  experimenting and reevaluating, 96–97, 111–12
  fast burners and, *see* Fast burners

Balance, The (cont.)
   flexibility of, 9–10, 71, 93
   goal of, 17
   ground rules, 97–101
   being prepared, 100–101
   breakfast, 97–98
   choosing best quality of foods possible, 101
   drinking water, 99
   eating five or six times a day, 98–99
   flour, wheat, and gluten, 99
   interchangeability of meal, 99–100
   stimulants, 97
   mixed burners and, see Mixed burners
   portion size and, 111
   pragmatism of, 92
   rewards of, 8–12, 29, 63, 82
   slow burners and, see Slow burners
Bananas, 122, 142
Bennet, William, 14
Beta-carotene, 70, 165
Beverages:
   for fast burners, 143, 144–45
   for slow burners, 123–24
Binges, 10, 65
Biochemical Individuality, 13
Biochemical individuality, xvi, 6, 13–14
BioPMT, 84
Bisson, Lionel, xv–xvii
Bland, Jeffrey, 163
Bloating, estrogen and, 83
Blood pressure:
   caffeine and, 55
   high, see High blood pressure
Blood sugar, 51, 62, 83
   see also Insulin
Blood types, 34–35
Body fat percentage, 130
Bowden, Jonathan, 96, 130–31

Brain, 67
   mental acuity and use of, 175
   sugar and, 63–65
   supplements to enhance mental function, 168, 174–75
Breakfast:
   eating, 97–98
   for fast burners, 141
   for slow burners, 125–26
Brigham and Women's Hospital, Boston, 106–107
Bulimia, 66, 74
Butter, 110

Caffeine, 48, 55, 57–58, 84, 123
   eliminating or reducing, 97
   see also Coffee
Calcitonin, 41
Calcium, 45, 86–87, 115
   slow burner and, 29
   supplements, 86–87
Cancer, 37
   reducing risk of, 12
   stress and, 47
Candida albicans, 174
Carbohydrates, 39, 67
   complex, 40, 64–65, 141
   simple, 40
   eliminating or reducing, 97
Cardiovascular disease, 8, 175
   supplements to promote cardiovascular health, 167, 175–76
Case studies:
   Eileen R., 148–49
   Frank, 11–12
   Phoebe L., 131–32
   Rhonda E., 86
   Roger W., 182–83
   Stan L., 93
   Susan, 11
   Susannah, 50–51
Catabolism, 6

Centers for Disease Control, 78
Chicken, 121, 140
Chinese restaurants, eating at, 128–29, 147
Chocolate, 83
Cholecystokinin (CCK), 51–52, 124
Cholesterol, xvii, 33
   elevated levels of, 38, 62
   fats and, 109–10
   HDL, 105, 109, 130
   LDL, 105, 109, 130
   trans fatty acids and, 105
Chronic fatigue, xvii, 48, 82
Chronic fatigue syndrome, 99
Cigarettes, see Tobacco
Citrus fruits, 122, 142
Clinical Nutrition Insights, 83
Coconut oil, 105
Coffee, 16, 49, 123
   decaffeinated, 55
   eliminating or reducing, 54–55, 97, 180
   see also Caffeine
Cold, sensitivity to, 117
Colgan Chronicles Newsletter, 170
Coliform bacteria, 173
Complex carbohydrates, 40, 64–65, 141
Compulsive behavior, 16
Concentration, 12, 48, 136
Cortisol, 41, 46, 51, 134, 135, 136
Cortisone, 109
Cranston, Dr. Elmer, 162
Cravings, 124, 137
   evolutionary reasons for, 32, 35, 60–61
   PMS and, 83
   supplements to control, 168
Criminal behavior, 66
Cro-Magnons, 34
Cytochrome P450 system, 162

Index

D'Adamo, Dr. Peter J., 34
Dairy products, 121, 140
Degenerative diseases, xvi, 37–38
  free radicals and, 69, 70
  stress and, 47
  see also specific diseases, e.g. Cancer; Heart disease
Deglycylrhizinate, 86
Depression, 5, 65, 66, 78
  mood enhancing supplements, 167, 172–73
Designer foods: shakes and power bars:
  for fast burners, 143
  for slow burners, 124
Design Protein, 124
Detoxification, 161–64
  supplements, 168
DeVore, Irven, 32
Diabetes, 38, 62
Diarrhea, 55
Diet, 180
  detoxification and, 161–62
  experimenting to find the right combination, 96–97
  for fast burners, see Fast burners, food plans for
  individual needs and, 95
  for mixed burners, 153–54
  quality of foods eaten, 101
  secret habits, 96
  for slow burners, see Slow burners, food plan for
  weight and, 94
Dieting, see Weight loss programs
Digestion, 12, 15
  chronic problems, 48
Dining out, see Restaurants, eating at
Dinner:
  for fast burners, 146
  for slow burners, 127–28
Distress, 45, 46
  see also Stress
Dizziness, 48
Docosahexaenoic acid (DHA), 106
"Do Diets Really Work?," 14
Dong quai, 85, 86
Drugs, 16, 48, 49
  prescription, see Prescription drugs
Dufty, William, 61, 62

East West Center for Holistic Health, xii, xiii
Eating disorders, 47, 66, 73–74
  see also Anorexia nervosa; Bulimia
Eating habits, see Diet
Eating out, see Restaurants, eating at
Eat Right for Your Type (D'Adamo), 34
Eczema, 47
Eggs, 109
Egyptians, 39
Eicosanoids, 107–108
Eicosapentaenoic acid (EPA), 106
Elavil, 66
Endorphins, 84
Endurance, 12
Energy enhancing supplements, 167, 171–72
Environment and metabolic type, 13
Ephedrine, 78
Equinox Training Institute, 96
Eskimos, 33, 102
Essential fatty acids (EFAs), 106–109
Estrogen, 87, 109
  PMS and, 83
Eustress, 46
  see also Stress
Exercise, 8, 92, 180, 181
  aerobic, see Aerobic exercise
  body fat percentage and, 130
  bones and, 87
  detoxification through, 162–63
  experimenting with, 96, 97
  fads, 8
  metabolic individualism and, 8
  for slow burners, 129–31
  stress reduction with, 84
  weight and, 94
  weight training, see Weight training

"Factory specification diet," 35–36
Fast burners, 6, 16, 17, 40, 133–49
  characteristics of, 29, 135–38
  physical conditions and diseases, 138
  psychological and physiological, 137
  evolution of, 38
  exercise for, 148
  fat storage by, 80–81
  food plan for, 138–43
    animal protein, 140
    beverages, 143
    designer foods: shakes and power bars, 143
    fats and oils, 142–43
    fruits, 142
    grains and grain products, 142
    vegetables, fibrous and starchy, 141
    vegetarian protein, 141
    percentage of, 133
  stress and, 49–50, 51
  structuring your day, 144–47
    bedtime snack, 147
    breakfast, 144–45
    eating out, 147

Fast burners (cont.)
lunch and dinner, 146
midmorning or midafternoon mini-meal, 145–46
sympathetic nervous system and, 41, 42
test to determine metabolic type, 17, 19–30
Fast food, 52
eating at fast-food chains, 129, 147
Fasts, water and juice, 162
Fatigue, 5, 135
chronic, *see* Chronic fatigue
energy enhancing supplements, 167, 171–72
"Fat on Thighs and Paunches Is the Fate of All Mammals," 80
Fats and oils, 32, 102–10
body's desire for, time between meals and, 98–99
body's storage of, 14–15, 80–81, 116–17
cholesterol and, 109–10
essential fatty acids, 106–109
for fast burners, 142–43
fat-free foods, 79, 102
monounsaturated, 104
polyunsaturated, 104
saturated, 103–105, 110
for slow burners, 123
toxin storage in body fat, 160
unsaturated, 103
Fenfluramine, 66–67
Fiber, 121
Fibrocystic disease, 55
Fight-or-flight response, 41, 45, 134
Fish, 121, 140
Flexibility, 9–10
Flippin, Royce, 129–30

Flour, 99
Fowkes, Steven, 165
Frackleton, Dr. James P., 162
Fraser, Laura, 76–7
Free radicals, 68–69, 162–63, 164–65
antioxidants and, 69–70
Fructose, 122
Fruit juices, 61, 123, 143
water and juice fasts, 162
Fruits:
for fast burners, 142
for slow burners, 122
tinned, 101

Galanin, 98
Gallbladder disease, 15
Gammalinoleic acid (GLA), 106
Genes, *see* Heredity
Gittleman, Ann Louise, 87, 105
Glucagon, 15, 115, 116, 122, 134
Glucose, 29, 61, 63
Gluten, 99
Gotu kola, 85, 86
Grains and grain products:
for fast burners, 142
for slow burners, 122–23
Greenwood, Dr. M. C. R., 80
Gurin, Joel, 14
Gurtmaker, Dr. Steven L., 74

Harvard School of Public Health, 74
Headaches, 5
migraine, *see* Migraine headaches
Health Nutrients (Quillin), 35–36
Health professionals, consulting, xix, 166, 169
Heart disease, 15, 33, 39, 62, 81
omega-3 oils and, 106

reducing risk of, 12
stress and, 47
Herbal supplements, *see* Supplements
Heredity:
evolution of metabolic types, 31–38
metabolic type and, 13
weight and, 94
High blood pressure, 47, 62, 81
High blood sugar, *see* Hyperglycemia
Hormonal imbalances, xvii
Hormone and hormone enhancing supplements, 168
Hormone replacement therapy (HRT), 85
Hot flashes, 85
Howell, Dr. Wanda, 110
"How Exercise Works," 129
Hunger, 9, 55
snacking to reduce, 99
see also Appetite
Hydrogenated vegetable oils, 105
Hyperglycemia, 51, 135
Hyperinsulinemia, 62, 116
Hypertension, 47, 62, 81
Hypoglycemia, 62, 83

Immune system:
strengthened, 12
sugar and, 60
supplements to boost, 167, 170–71
Individuality, xvii, 13
biochemical, *see* Biochemical individuality
diet and, 95
of stress reaction, 44, 47
Insomnia, 48, 55, 117
Insulin, 61–62, 63, 65, 115, 116, 122, 134
cholesterol production and, 110
distribution of essential fatty acids and, 109
Insulin resistance, 62–63

Index

Insurance company weight tables, 76–77
Intestines:
  filtering of toxins by, 159, 160
  problems with, xvii
Involuntary nervous system, 41, 114, 116, 134
  balance in, 114–15
  parasympathetic nervous system, *see* Parasympathetic nervous system
  sympathetic nervous system, *see* Sympathetic nervous system
Irritability, 48, 55, 135
ISO powder, 124
Italian restaurants, eating at, 129, 147

Journal of Holistic Medicine, 162

Kelley, William, 19
Kidneys, filtering of toxins by, 159
Krohn, Dr. Jacqueline, 60

Lactobacillus acidophilus, 173
Lemonick, Michael, 66
Life, 73–74
Life Extension Foundation, 166
Lifestyles, healthy living and stressed, 4–5
Lighten Up: Food, Weight and Self-Image, 75
Linoleic acid, 106
Linolenic acid, 106
Lipoprotein lipase (LPL), 14, 81
Liquid diets, 78
Liquor, *see* Alcohol
Liver, filtering of toxins by, 159, 161
Longevity:
  anti-aging supplements, 167, 176
  antioxidants and, 164–66
  science of health and, 157–83
  Losing It: America's Obsession with Weight and the Industry That Feeds on It (Fraser), 76–77
Lowey, Nita, 74
Lunch:
  for fast burners, 146
  for slow burners, 127–28
Lupus, 82

McNamara, Dr. Donald, 110
Magnesium, 45, 83
  slow burner and, 29
Margarine, 105, 110
Mayo, Dr. Joseph L., 83, 84
Meals:
  eating five or six times a day, 98–99
  interchangeability of, 99–100
  see also Breakfast; Dinner; Lunch
Meat eaters, evolution of, 33
Meats, red, 105–106, 109, 121, 140
Medicine, *see* Prescription drugs
Men and fats, 80
Menopause, 85–86
Menstrual cramps, 12
Mental function, supplements to enhance, 168, 174–75
Metabolic individuality, 6, 7, 13–14, 39, 92
  becoming balanced burner within your type, 29
  determinants of, 13
  evolution of, 31–38
  exercise and, 8
  fast burners, *see* Fast burners
  identifying your metabolic type, 17, 19–30
  learning to work with what you've got, 93–94
  mixed burners, *see* Mixed burners
  slow burners, *see* Slow burners
  test to determine your type, 17, 19–30
Metabolism, 135
  The Balance, *see* Balance, The
  defined, 6
  fast burners, *see* Fast burners
  individuality of, *see* Metabolic individuality
  mixed burners, *see* Mixed burners
  negative effects of unbalanced, 30
  slow burners, *see* Slow burners
  supplements to enhance, 168, 169–70
  understanding your, xvi
Metabolites, 162
Metagenics, 163
Mexican restaurants, eating at, 129, 147
Migraine headaches, xi–xii, xiii, xvii, 47, 59, 66, 179–80
Mineral supplements, *see individual minerals*; Supplements
Mixed burners, 6, 17, 40, 151–55
  characteristics of, 29, 152–53
  evolution of, 38
  exercise for, 155
  food plan for, 153–54
  sympathetic and parasympathetic nervous systems and, 114
  test to determine metabolic type, 17, 19–30

Monounsaturated fats, 104
Mood enhancing supplements, 167, 172–73
Mood swings, xvii, 5, 12, 58, 134
Muscle building supplements, 168
Muscle Media, 170

National Health and Nutrition Examination Survey, 37
Neck pain, 48
Neolithic man, 34
Nervous system, 114
 see also Involuntary nervous system; Voluntary nervous system
New York magazine, xvi
New York Times, 79, 80
Next Nutrition, 124
NPD, 79
Nutritional information, 5
 bombardment with, xvii, 4, 95, 158
 contradictory, xvii, 96
Nutritional needs, *see* Diet

Obesity, xvii, 37, 39, 62
Obsessive-compulsive disorder, 66
Oils, *see* Fats and oils
Olestra, 79
Omega-3 fatty acids, 106–107
Omega-6 fatty acids, 106
Optimal Nutrition Review (South), 64
Oral contraceptives, 174
Osteoporosis, 82, 86–87
Overeating, 16, 48, 66

Pancreas, 40, 41, 61, 115, 116
Panic attacks, 55
Parasympathetic nervous system, 40, 41, 42, 115, 134, 151–52
 balance with sympathetic nervous system, 114

Parathyroid gland, 115
Parathyroid glands, 40
Pear-shaped body type, 81, 117
Phentermine, 66–67
Phosphate, 115
Physician, consulting your, xix, 166, 169
Physiology of Stress, The, 134
PMS, *see* Premenstrual syndrome (PMS)
Polyunsaturated fats, 104
Potassium, 32, 122, 142
 slow burner and, 28–29
Power bars, 124, 143
"Premenstrual Syndrome: A Natural Approach to Management," 83, 99
Premenstrual syndrome (PMS), 5, 12, 48, 66, 82–85
 supplements for, 84–85
Preparedness, 100–101
Prescription drugs, 66–67, 78
 caution for persons taking, xix
Preservatives, 37, 70
Pritikin, Nathan, 102, 103
Pritikin diet, 103
Processed and refined foods, 37, 38, 49, 69, 101
Procter & Gamble, 79
Protein, *see* Animal protein; Vegetarian protein
Prozac, 66
Psychological therapy, 67
Psychology Today, 73, 75
Purine-rich proteins, 141

Quillin, Dr. Patrick, 35–36

Redux (dexfenfluramine), 66–67
Refined foods, *see* Processed and refined foods

Relaxation, 136
Resources guide, 189–91
Restaurants, eating at, 71
 fast burners, 147
 flexibility when, 9–10
 slow burners, 158–59
Root vegetables, 70

Saffron, Dr. Sidney, xiii–xiv
St. John's wort, 85, 132, 173
Saturated fats, 103–105, 110
Saunas, 163
Scheibel, Dr. Arnold, 175
Schizophrenia, 66
Science, 14
Sears, Dr. Barry, xvi, 108
Seasonal foods, 101
Self, 129
Selye, Dr. Hans, 45, 54
Serotonin, 65–66, 67, 173
Sex, diminished interest in, 5
Shakes, 124
 for fast burners, 143
 Ultra Clear, 163–64
Silverstein, Dr. Brett, 77
Silverstone, Alicia, 76
Skin:
 aging and, 164–65
 filtering of toxins by, 160
Sleep problems,
 see Insomnia
Slow burners, 6, 16–17, 40, 113–32
 characteristics of, 28–29, 115–19
 physical conditions and disease, 118–19
 psychological and physiological, 117–18
 evolution of, 38
 exercise for, 129–31
 food plan for, 119–24
  animal protein, 121
  beverages, 123–24
  designer foods: shakes and power bars, 124

fats and oils, 123
fruits, 122
grains and grain products, 122–23
vegetables, fibrous and starchy, 121–22
vegetarian protein, 121
parasympathetic nervous system and, 41
percentage of, 113
stress and, 51
structuring your day, 125–29
bedtime snack, 128
breakfast, 125–26
eating out, 128–29
lunch and dinner, 127–28
midmorning of midafternoon minimeal, 126–27
test to determine metabolic type, 17, 19–30
Smart Drug News, 165
Smart Exercise (Bailey), 163
Smoking, *see* Tobacco
Snacks, 98–99
for fast burners, 145–46, 147
for slow burners, 126–27, 128
Sodium, 32
cravings for, 35
slow burner and, 28–29
Soft drinks, 124, 143
South, James, 64
Soy products:
for fast burners, 141
for slow burners, 121
Steam baths, 163
Stress, 43–56
ability to cope with, 12, 47, 49–50
defined, 44
disease and, 44, 47
distress versus eustress, 46

evolution of stress response, 48–49
food and, 50–52
free radicals and, 164, 165
general adaptation syndrome (GAS), 45–48
individuality of, 44
PMS and, 84
stages of, 44–48
test, 52–54
warning signs, 47–48
Stress of Life, The (Selye), 46
Sugar, 37, 40, 49, 54, 58–65, 83, 174
blood sugar, *see* Blood sugar
the brain and, 63–65
children and, 58–59
cravings for, 32, 60–61
eliminating or reducing, 97
in fat-free foods, 79
PMS and cravings for, 83
Sugar Blues (Dufty), 61, 62
Sunlight and depression, 173
Supermetabolism, xiv, 29, *see also* Balance, The
Super Nutrition for Women (Gittleman), 87
Supplements, 7–8, 158–59, 166–76, 181
anti-aging, 167, 176
antioxidants, 70, 167
for cardiovascular health, 167
caution about taking, xix
for craving control, 168
detoxifiers, 168
energy enhancers, 167, 171–72
experimenting with combinations of, 169
glossary of, 187–88
hormones and hormone enhancers, 168
for immunity/risk prevention, 167, 170–71
intelligent use of, 166–69

mood enhancers, 167, 172–73
muscle builders, 168
for PMS, 84–85
smart nutrients/brain boosters, 168, 174–75
weight management/metabolic enhancers, 168, 169–70
Sweating and elimination of toxins, 162–63
Sweets, 59 *see also* Sugar
Sympathetic nervous system, 40, 41, 42, 45, 115, 134, 151–52
balance with parasympathetic nervous system, 114

Taylor, Elizabeth, 76
Tea, 123–24
Teeth, 39
grinding of, 48
Testosterone, 109
Tests:
to determine metabolic type, 17, 19–30
stress, 52–54
Thermogenics, 169–70
Thompson, Kevin, 75
Thorne Research, 84
Thyroid gland, 40, 41, 51, 115, 134, 135
Time, 66
Tinned foods, 101
Tobacco, 16, 48, 49, 54, 84, 97, 160
Townsend Letter for Patients and Doctors, 170
Toxins, 159–64
body's filtering systems, 159–60
consequences of toxic overload, 161
defined, 160
detoxification, 161–64
Trace Elements and Other Essential Nutrients (Watts), 45, 47, 117

Index

Trans fatty acids, 105, 110
Triglycerides, 33
Tropical fruits, 37
Turkey, 121, 140
Type AB blood type, 34
Type A blood type, 34
Type A personality, 16, 42, 135
Type B blood type, 34
Type B personality, 42

Ulcers, 47
Ultra Clear, 163–64
Unsaturated fats, 103

Vegetables:
 for fast burners, 141
 for slow burners, 121–22
 tinned, 111
Vegetarian diet, xiii
 evolution of, 33, 38
Vegetarian protein:
 for fast burners, 141
 for slow burners, 121
Violent crime, 66
Vitamin B12, 33
Vitamin C, 60–61, 70, 165
 cravings for, 35
Vitamin D, 109
Vitamin D3, 87
Vitamin E, 70, 165
Vitamin supplements, *see individual vitamins;* Supplements
Voluntary nervous system, 114

Wall Street Journal, 32
Warm, tendency to feel, 136

Water, 123, 143
 fasts, juice and, 162
Water, drinking, 99
Watts, Dr. David, 19, 45, 47, 117
Weight:
 body fat percentage, 130
 factors determining your, 94
 healthy for you, 82
 losing, *see* Weight loss; Weight loss programs
 maintaining stable, 12
 set point, 82
 supplements for weight management, 168, 169–70
 women and, *see* Women and weight
Weight gain, 117, 136
Weight loss:
 desire for, 5
 men and, 80
 program for, *see* Weight loss programs
 regaining lost weight, 14–15
 supplements for, 168, 169–70
Weight loss programs:
 individuality, ignoring, 6–7
 money spent on, 4, 78–80
 yo-yo-dieting, 14–15
Weight training, 8, 148, 163
Wheat, 99
Whey peptide beverages, 124
Whole Way to Allergy Relief and Prevention, The (Krohn), 60
Williams, Dr. Roger J., xvi, 13–14, 19
Women and weight, 73–82
 body image, 73–74, 75, 81
 food industry and, 79–80
 food preparation, responsibility for, 78
 healthy weight for you, 82
 history of, 76–77
 Hot Seat exercise, 75
 impact of being overweight, 74, 77–78
 storage of fat, 80–81
 thinness versus well-being, 76
Women and Weight program, 75
Women's health, 82–87
Women's News, 74

Yankelovich Partners, 70–71
Yeast, overgrowth of, 173–74
Yeast infections, 99
Your Body Knows Best (Gittleman), 105
Yo-yo-dieting, 14–15

Zone, The (Sears), xvi, 108